Dealing With Anxiety And Panic

Arm Yourself With Information, Relieve Anxiety, Prevent Panic Attacks, Know How To Care And What Remedies To Use

ISBN-13: 978-1721054701

ISBN-10: 1721054707

Legal & Disclaimer

The information contained in this book and its contents is not designed to replace or take the place of any form of medical or professional advice; and is not meant to replace the need for independent medical, financial, legal or other professional advice or services, as may be required. The content and information in this book have been provided for educational and entertainment purposes only.

The content and information contained in this book have been compiled from sources deemed reliable, and it is accurate to the best of the Author's knowledge, information, and belief. However, the Author cannot guarantee its accuracy and validity and cannot be held liable for any errors and/or omissions. Further, changes are periodically made to this book as and when needed. Where appropriate and/or necessary, you must consult a professional (including but not limited to your doctor, attorney, financial advisor or such other professional advisor) before using any of the suggested remedies, techniques, or information in this book.

Contents

PART 1: INTRODUCTION

1.0 INTRODUCTION

Everyone gets worried sometimes; we all wonder what tomorrow holds. Students wonder whether they'll will finish school with the grades they dreamt of, women hope that they will one day become wives and mothers, teenagers fret over meeting timelines set by society; generally, we are anxious about the uncertainty of our lives. The fear of the unknown keeps us second-guessing ourselves every day. This is not abnormal; worrying is what makes us human. However, when this worry begins to control us, begins to affect our everyday lives, makes us paranoid and lasts for over 6 months, it has become a disorder and it is time to get help. The funny thing about this is that there might really be nothing to worry about; we just spend so much time and emotion on nothing. In every attempt, we make to achieve more goals in life, we usually see and focus on the negativities and this causes us to achieve little or nothing.

Are you tired of experiencing numb feet and fingers, sweaty nights, insomnia and other tiresome occurrences? Is your friend, spouse, mother, father, sibling or anyone close to you suffering from uneasiness, heart palpitations and other symptoms associated with anxiety and/or panic? Does this worry you? Have you been confusing anxiety with depression? Do you feel uninformed about anxiety and panic disorders? Do you feel alone in your situation or that your close one is the only patient with these disorders? Are you at a loss as to how to go about treating the disorders? Do you wonder what steps to follow to get the cure you or your loved one deserves?

If you answered yes to any of the above questions, then you should proceed with digesting the subsequent chapters of this book. *Dealing with Panic and Anxiety* approaches disorders in a way that most books do not. The book presents researchers' view of what anxiety and panic are and what the possible causes and symptoms may be. It also provides some comfort and hope to patients or their close ones that they are not alone, that there are those who have successfully overcome their disorders, that there is light at the end of the tunnel. It does not leave you hanging, no; it provides possible ways to avoid getting into that boat at all and for those who are already there, a systematic guide on how to get treatment through natural means, medication, therapy and self-help.

The author hopes that after reading this book, women facing anxiety and panic disorders or their close ones will not only have a better understanding of what these conditions are and how they come to be, but also how to overcome them and make sure that they remain in the past. We expect that after reading this book, women will learn to live life fully by accepting life for what it is (imperfect and dynamic) and not keel themselves over for not meeting some flimsy societal standard. We are hopeful that by the time you finish reading this book, you will learn to accept the things you cannot change, twist negative situations into good ones and help others survive anxiety and panic.

1.1 ANXIETY

Anxiety is the general term for extreme feelings of nervousness and panic, which worsen overtime. Once the anxious feeling becomes aggravated, irrational, haunting, uncontrollable, and interferes with a person's daily life, it has developed into an anxiety disorder and requires attention.

Anxiety as a disorder that does not just pop up in a person's life, it is traceable to a series of risk factors associated with the patient and certain symptoms must have been exhibited before the disorder comes to be.

Research shows that women are twice as likely to suffer from anxiety disorders than men are. This is possibly because women are generally more emotional than men are and most women worry more about societal acceptance than some men do.

Whatever the reason may be, anxiety disorders are not a pleasant experience for either the sufferers and their close ones. Therefore, good knowledge of preventative measures, causes and the symptoms is important in order to keep the disorder in check or avoid it altogether.

1.2 PANIC

Some people think that panic disorders or panic attacks are a type of anxiety disorder and the two should be treated the same. The "Diagnostic and Statistical Manual of Mental Disorders, 5th edition," known as the DSM-5, uses the term *panic attack* to describe the hallmark features associated with the condition known as panic disorder, so they support the notion that panic disorders are their own phenomenon.

It is a sudden dominating feeling of fear, terror or anxiety, which is so strong that it blocks flow of logical, rational reasoning and action. It envelopes the body, taking over the hormones and entire being of the person experiencing it; it could result in a near-death experience because a person's breath could seize too. It happens at random. People experience panic attacks once or twice in a lifetime but if it becomes a recurrent thing, it is a disorder.

Panic attacks happen in three dimensions:

- Intense: The feeling of a gun being held to your head. It overwhelms you and usually precedes a feeling of impending doom which leaves you petrified of another such attack.
- Sudden: It comes without warning and often forcefully. In cases like this, a person is either upset about an event or anxious about an anticipated occurrence.
- Panic Waves: These come often with intense fright. It comes in waves until a "safe place" has been located and the person has occupied it. It leaves the person drained both physically and emotionally.

Panic can be said to be more dangerous than anxiety because it can occur at any time and without warning; while driving a car, while piloting a plane, during an interview, in your sleep, literally at any time. As if that isn't bad enough, it peaks within minutes and could last for an hour. The good news is that treatment is very effective.

1.3 ANXIETY VS. DEPRESSION

It is common for most individuals suffering from depression to assume they have an anxiety disorder. This is common even among medical practitioners and it is excusable because both psychological issues have some similarities in symptoms and there is an overlap in the treatment procedure. While this is common, it is almost impossible to cure anxiety successfully by administering treatments for depression; in fact in some cases, it could be fatal or counter-productive.

While depression is a melancholic feeling of severe dejection, sadness or worthlessness, which affects a person's behavior and attitude towards others as well as how a person handles issues in their life, anxiety is as explained in the preceding paragraphs of this chapter.

Symptoms of depression include loss of interest in enjoyable activities, lack of concentration, suicidal thoughts, feelings of worthlessness, sluggishness, increased or decreased appetite, etc. and which symptoms must go on for about two weeks to qualify as a disorder. However, symptoms of anxiety as discussed in the next part of this book are required to persist for a period of six months to be diagnosed as a disorder.

More differences are:

- While anxiety causes someone to want to escape from all the negative occurrences around them, depression suggests suicide.
- Depression is certainty that nothing positive is likely to happen, anxiety is uncertainty that everything will go smoothly.
- Depression makes a person less likely to move as they have no energy and feel that nothing can change the certain bad future, but anxiety patients usually

experience sweating, shaking and readiness to run should the expected negative event happen.

While the two are highly similar and anxiety can lead to depression, it is imperative to understand the differences in order to administer adequate treatment.

1.4 PANIC VS. FEAR

Just as depression is often mistaken for anxiety, mere fear and panic are often mistaken for each other and this isn't accurate either. Panic draws from fear in that extreme fear culminates in panic. While fear is a normal, general human feeling, Panic is a cause for concern because it is an anomaly.

Some basic differences between the two are:

- While fear is anticipatory, panic is instant, in other words, it occurs during the fright-inducing event.
- While fear activates survival tactics, for instance the fight or flight response, panic activates sweating, shivering, and a feeling of dread.
- When fear occurs, there is rapid breathing, a surge of adrenaline and the like, but with panic, the person is hardly able to determine what physical reactions take place until after he or she must have calmed down.
- Fear is a rational response to situations that threaten our safety, while panic can be irrational.
- Panic can be a progressive or heightened form of anxiety; in other words, it is a consequence of anxiety but fear is not - it is not a consequence of a disorder.
- Panic attacks could happen in a person's sleep and could last for up to an hour, but fear requires knowledge that something is about to occur and happens mostly when the individual is awake and in their full senses.
- Even though panic is a disorder deserving immediate attention, fear should be addressed because it could cause a negative effect on the scared individual if not properly controlled; for instance, a scared person might freeze in the face of anticipatory danger or in an attempt to flee, would run in the direction of danger.

PART 2: RESEARCH AND FINDINGS

Here, we look at a summary of the conclusions drawn by researchers on the causes, symptoms and types of anxiety disorders and those of panic disorders. These come from a plethora of sources and are put together in simple terms, leaving out the details of scientific experiments and philosophical theories in order to make things more comprehensible for you.

2.0 CAUSES OF ANXIETY

In treating anxiety, understanding the cause is a major step and that is what makes this section important. Anxiety disorder is not necessarily a decision a person makes; no sane person consciously decides to experience it. Varieties of factors that cause anxiety disorder are mostly traceable to the environment, lifestyle, family, experiences and medical history of the patient. The categories of causes are *medical causes* and *risk factors* (which could be both internal and external factors).

MEDICAL CAUSES

There are certain situations that would require a doctor to conduct some medical tests to ascertain whether the anxiety is a disorder that has occurred on its own, is drawn from an underlying medical disease or is a side effect from the use of a medication. The causes that fall within these three categories are what researchers refer to as medical causes.

Being a medical cause does not necessarily mean that the solutions will involve the prescription of medication. For instance, withdrawal from the drug may treat anxiety caused by drug abuse, and psychotherapy without any medication can help too.

The medical causes include:

- Rare tumors which produce certain fight-or-flight hormones

- Menopause
- Seizures
- Withdrawal from alcohol, anti-anxiety medications (Benzodiazepines) or other medications
- Mental retardation
- Thyroid problems like hyperthyroidism
- Mitral Valve Prolapse
- Respiratory disorders, such as Chronic Obstructive Pulmonary Disease (COPD) and asthma
- Prostate cancer
- Diabetes
- Drug misuse
- Heart disease
- Chronic pain or IBS (Irritable Bowel Syndrome)
- Chemical imbalance: an imbalance of certain neurotransmitters like serotonin, norepinephrine and gamma-aminobutyric acid (GABA) has been discovered to be a major cause of anxiety.

RISK FACTORS

In either childhood or infancy, there are experiences that a person may encounter that could bring about anxiety disorder. It could also occur due to the medical history of the family (hereditary factors) and trigger anxious feelings that might metamorphose into a disorder. The painful thing about risk factors is that the person may not be able to do anything to avoid experiencing them because sometimes, they are born with them. Nevertheless, the good thing is that when they grow up or after the traumatizing event, they can make the choice to be free of the effects of a painful childhood or bad experience by choosing happiness and refusing to let anxiety control them.

Some risk factors are:

- **Personality:** Those with certain personality types (e.g. melancholic) are more prone to suffer anxiety disorders than others (e.g. sanguine) are. People who fall under the melancholic temperament are prone to pessimism and are generally anxious about the future. When faced with a situation, they first see all the existing factors for why it won't work out, then they analyze how impossible it is to avoid these factors and the fear of failure brings about anxious feelings, which may metamorphose into an anxiety attack.

- **Change:** Strange as it may seem, change (albeit positive) can cause anxiety in a person. A new job, home, environment, promotion, or even marriage can cause anxiety in the person experiencing the change. Most times, the anxious feeling comes from the fear of imperfection; the new wife or employee begins to see all the things she can do that may cause her to make a mess of her new position. Now that the likely mistakes are known, instead of dwelling on all the things she can do to ensure that she does not make those mistakes, an anxious person dwells on all the bad things that could happen when she makes those mistakes. This leads to an anxiety attack and if it becomes recurrent, an anxiety disorder.

- **Stress induced by illness:** Serious health conditions, especially terminal illnesses, can cause significant worry about issues like the unlikelihood of a cure, what the future holds and how the people they leave behind when they die will survive. A practical person will most likely begin to set up structures to mitigate the problems that could arise out of her death; for instance, writing a valid will to solve inheritance issues, but an anxious person will analyze the problems associated with dying instead, think of how the problems may destroy her family and subsequently suffer an anxiety attack.

- **Accumulated Stress:** An accumulation of smaller, stressful life situations, for example the death of a family member or loved one, stress from work, or ongoing worries about finances and other life situations may bring about excessive anxiety. It is okay to worry, but it is wrong to make it the order of the day. Excessive worry is one of the causes of anxiety.

- **Anxiety:** It may be weird, but an anxious feeling about certain things, like a first boat ride, can cause future anxiety over boat rides. This also applies to having a negative thought or previous experience of symptoms of anxiety. Therefore, (using the instance of a boat ride) every time it is time to travel by water or every time a person thinks of a boat ride, they experience the symptoms related to anxiety and then comes the attack. People in this situation are encouraged to overcome the fear by successfully engaging in that anxiety causing activity continuously.

- **Trauma:** People who experienced abuse or trauma during their growing years or any time in their past are more prone to suffer anxiety disorders at some stage in their lives than those who had a happy childhood. For people who suffered trauma, it is important to see a shrink immediately after a traumatic event so that the healing process can begin.

- **Genetics:** Anxiety disorders could be hereditary such that if a person has a family member who has suffered or is suffering from an anxiety disorder, chances are that they would experience it too. While we cannot choose the families we are born into, we can decide what we make of the unfortunate things we inherit from our progenitors. A person with a family history of anxiety disorder should not wait for the first attack before seeking help, a healthy lifestyle and regular visits to the doctor can help prevent or cure the hereditary anxiety.

- **Emotional Stress:** Pain or trauma from a failed relationship, crisis in a marriage or long-term disagreement between family members or friends can cause extreme anxiety. "No one is worth the stress" is a popular saying among tough girls. This does not mean that you shouldn't feel bad when your relationship with others begins to go south, but rather than worry, why not do something to salvage it?

- **Drugs or Alcohol Abuse and Addiction:** The use of, misuse of or withdrawal from drugs and alcohol can trigger or worsen anxiety in the persons involved. While some alcohol is good for the body, too much of it can cause both anatomical and psychological harm. Some researchers see drug abuse as inherently bad and withdrawal from both is not an easy process. The most rational thing to do here is seek help from professionals or even survivors of the abuse and addiction to drugs and alcohol.
- **Pregnancy:** During pregnancy, women usually experience hormonal imbalances that cause mood swings, strange and epileptic appetites and cravings, etc. Pregnant women also worry about things as little as the temperature of the water they drink to big things like being a great mother or having a safe delivery. If anxiety develops at pregnancy, it may be difficult to diagnose it as a disorder and so by the time it is realized, it may be too late. For instance, pregnancy lasts for 9 months, a woman who started showing signs of anxiety in the first trimester will be a full patient of anxiety disorder by the time she gives birth if nothing was done about it. Worse still, this could affect the baby in the womb too. Thus, it is important to regularly check and monitor anxiety during pregnancy, not dismiss it as normal.
- **Other Psychological Disorders:** People with other psychological disorders, such as depression and panic, often also have an anxiety disorder. In cases like this, treating only anxiety may not cure it, it is important to find the underlying cause of the anxiety and solve the problem at its roots.
- **Environment:** Shortage of oxygen is a major characteristic of high altitudes; a person who finds him or herself in such an environment can experience anxiety too. Those who know that they cannot endure such an environment should either go there with the necessary protective items (for example; an oxygen mask) or avoid visiting such places altogether.

2.1 SYMPTOMS OF ANXIETY

The fundamental symptoms of this disorder start out as normal day-to-day reactions to problems, like normal worries or nervousness about a debt, a missing item, a job interview, or even normal symptoms of mild illnesses. It is after some period of observation that one realizes that they have been displaying these symptoms repeatedly over a long period (usually six months) and realizes that something isn't right.

The Anxiety Disorders Association of America states that women are twice as likely as men to suffer from anxiety disorders such as anxiety attacks. Therefore, these symptoms are more noticeable in women. It is worse for women too because some of these symptoms like irritability, cramps, nausea, or dizziness are also symptoms of normal physiological and anatomical developments like ovulation, menstruation, pregnancy and menopause, and so the symptoms could go on being misunderstood until it is too late. The symptoms include:

- Cold sweats
- Numb or tingling feet and fingers
- Heart palpitations
- Dry Mouth
- Lack of sleep
- Shortness of breath
- Nausea
- Uneasiness
- Excessive fear
- Irritability
- Dizziness
- Obsessive thinking or worrying

It is worthy to note that the above symptoms are not particularly unique to anxiety, as other psychological disorders like depression and panic also enjoy similar symptoms; even if this had not been the case, self-diagnosis techniques, like self-medication, is wrong. For these reasons, you must bear in mind that these symptoms do not necessarily negate the need for a diagnosis and it is therefore important to see a doctor in order to determine the exact type of disorder one has and dispense the proper treatment.

2.2 TYPES OF ANXIETY DISORDERS

Anxiety is the general name for different psychological conditions that involve fear and worry. So beyond having an anxiety disorder, it is important to determine what type of anxiety disorder the patient is suffering from in order to administer the right form of treatment, because a misdiagnosis could lead to wrong treatment and ultimately worsen the condition. There are fundamentally seven known types of anxiety disorders:

1. General Anxiety Disorder (GAD): This is the most rampant type of anxiety disorder. A recurrent state of mental tension, physical tension, and nervousness, which is probably linkable to a specific source or is involuntary.
   So essentially, constant physical or mental stress, edginess and worry that disrupts everyday life and affects the way life issues are approached point towards GAD. A person who suffers from this will need to consult a specialist to be sure and to get adequate treatment as soon as possible.
   A variety of factors can bring about GAD including perfectionist tendencies, a breakdown in an otherwise successful relationship, and changes in brain function, as well as family history.

2. Specific Phobias: In this case, due to a previous bad experience; a person might begin to be quite fearful of an object, an animal or an activity, like travelling in a plane, receiving injections, swimming, a lion, a spider, etc.
   Some people react to the phobic stimulus (subject of fear) by merely imagining it or seeing a picture or watching it on TV. Most people who have this kind of

fear are aware of the irrationality but feel that it is impossible to control or stop the feeling.

Persons with this phobia may experience panic attacks, faintness, nausea, choking, and cold flushes.

3. <u>Panic Disorders:</u> This is extreme fear, worry or a feeling of doom that something is about to go wrong or is actually wrong. For instance, getting a bed space in a hospital on the insistence that all is not well with their health. This is traceable to the symptoms associated with the disorder, like headaches, chest pain, digestive problems, shortness of breath, ear pressure, stomach pain, depersonalization, dizziness, excessive perspiration, etc. All these symptoms are very real.

Persistent panic attacks mostly characterize the disorder, as well as the fear of having panic attacks, either of which goes on for about a month. Some of those experiencing a panic attack usually think it is a heart attack until it is over.

4. <u>Obsessive Compulsive Disorder (OCD):</u> Here, a person has certain fears that they may consider silly but which pushes them to execute certain actions as measures to prevent the cause of fear. A ready example is constant use of hand sanitizers induced by fear of germs. So, a person with this disorder constantly carries out activities to neutralize the negative thought or alleviate distress, thus they are seen always trying to make sure that there is no cause for alarm by making sure that everything is in perfect condition and in their rightful place.

Persons with this condition experience a delay in diagnosis sometimes because some of them are usually ashamed and often try to hide their compulsions, this can worsen into social disability as they begin to avoid people.

Some symptoms include cleanliness, hoarding, accuracy, counting, religious or moral issues (praying too often), perfectionism, etc.

5. <u>Social Phobia:</u> Also known as social anxiety, social phobia manifests in public places. Some level of shyness in public is okay, but when it becomes so bad as to cause fear of socializing and interferes with the daily routine of the affected individual, then social phobia is imminent and immediate help is advisable.

The symptoms include severe fear of public speaking, obsessing over being watched, worrying about doing something stupid in public, anxiety about the 'idea' of a social situation without necessarily being in one, feeling hopeless among strangers, etc.

The situation is so bad that they are extremely nervous about meeting strangers, public speaking, eating in public, exchanging ideas in a formal setting, etc. It could also be specific if the person is not generally nervous about partaking in social functions but about getting involved in a particular social function.

6. <u>Agoraphobia:</u> Agoraphobia is the fear of open spaces or unfamiliar locations. Persons with this condition often prefer to remain indoors, avoid travelling and often restrict themselves to familiar routes and environments.

For some people, it comes after having a panic attack, for others it is due to fear of losing control in public. It is most common in adults. The symptoms include tension or stress when engaging in outdoor activities, obsessive fear of socialization, severe anxiety in unfamiliar environments, irrational fear of confined places, fear of using public transportation, etc.

7. <u>Post-Traumatic Stress Disorder (PTSD):</u> As the name suggests, it is the psychological stress experienced after a traumatic event has occurred in one's life. It is so serious that failure to seek help could cause it to continue for years after the event has occurred, or even for the rest of a person's life. It is both physical and psychological and both the person who experienced the

event first-hand and in some cases, the person who witnessed another person's experience of a traumatic event, suffer from the disorder.

Some symptoms are reliving the trauma (flashbacks), emotional detachment, anxiety over a recurrence of the event, upsetting dreams, nightmares, etc. Some traumatic experiences include war, sexual assault, witnessing murder, kidnap, physical assault, accidents, and natural disaster.

Where the PTSD has continued for a long period, other problems begin to show up, like anxiety, depression, alcohol abuse, use of hard drugs, paranoia, etc. We recommend immediate help for persons facing this challenge.

Determining the particular type of anxiety disorder is a bit tricky, so researchers and therapies have organized some tests taken by patients to determine the type of anxiety disorder they are suffering from. In addition, a person may suffer from more than one anxiety disorder at a time. For instance, traces of General Anxiety Disorder (GAD) may also exist in persons suffering from a panic disorder or Obsessive Compulsive Disorder.

2.3 CAUSES OF PANIC

Even though panic happens suddenly and randomly, it is traceable to many factors. Here, we shall discuss the causes of panic as they relate to the disorder. Different people have different reasons for panicking and because of these diverse reasons, the direct causes of panic are unknown. Nevertheless, researchers have traced and classified some factors into medical causes and risk factors (internal and external).

MEDICAL CAUSES

- Certain changes in brain function
- Genetics
- Stress-sensitive or pessimistic temperaments
- Major stress

RISK FACTORS

This refers to certain factors, which can occur in a person's life at birth, early childhood, adolescence, or even adulthood that may increase the chances of having panic attacks and lead to panic disorders. They are:

- Family history of panic attacks or panic disorders.
- A past traumatic event, like physical or sexual assault, disaster or accidents.
- Major changes in life, like a divorce, a break-up or a new baby.
- Excessive consumption of caffeine.
- History of physical or sexual abuse.

2.4 SYMPTOMS OF PANIC DISORDERS

The symptoms of panic include:

- Hyperventilation
- Headache
- Apprehension of doom
- Faintness
- Abdominal cramping
- Dizziness
- Fear of loss of control or death
- Chest pain
- Rapid heartrate or heart Palpitations
- Sweating
- Lightheadedness
- Trembling or shaking
- Fear of death
- Chills
- Tightness in the throat
- Phobic avoidance (avoiding places and circumstances that may cause panic)
- Hot or cold flashes
- Nausea
- Paresthesia (Numbness or tingling sensation)
- Feeling of unreality or detachmentIf these symptoms persist beyond a month, or the panic attacks persist for as long, it is imperative to visit a psychologist.

2.5 TYPES OF PANIC ATTACKS AND DISORDERS

There are fundamentally four types of Clinical Panic Disorders we know of:

- Type I: The only symptom is a single panic attack.
- Type II: Here, panic attacks occur oftentimes but without any accompanying neurotic or depressive symptoms.
- Type III: There is a recurrence of panic attacks accompanied by gradual development of neurotic symptoms, like agoraphobia, generalized anxiety, anticipatory anxiety, or hypochondriasis.
- Type IV: Panic attacks recur but with depressive symptoms. Type IV is further divided into three subtypes:
  - Type IV-1: At this level, the depressive symptoms develop incidental to panic attacks and subsequently, major depression coexists with the panic disorder.
  - Type IV-2: The panic disorder constantly progresses into major depression.
  - Type IV-3: Things are now apparent; the panic attacks as well as depressive symptoms exist independently.

The most common types are Type III and Type IV-1, and seem to be a core group of the panic disorder.

There are three types of panic disorders (or attacks). They are:

- **Uncued (Unexpected) Panic Attacks:** Some psychologists refer to these as "Out of the blue" panic attacks because they are spontaneous and there might be no defined cause. The recurrence of this type of panic attack is a basis for panic disorder.
- **Cued (Situational) Panic Attacks:** This occurs in anticipation of a triggering event. For instance, a person with a specific phobia of flying can experience a panic attack every time she thinks of travelling by air). In this case, the cause is traceable.

- **Situationally Predisposed Panic Attacks:** This category shares similarities with cued panic attacks, but they are not always linkable to a cue, nor do they invariably occur immediately after exposure to the causes. In other words, a person could go through the panic-inducing activity without experiencing panic and may not have any such attack until long after engaging in the activity.

PART 3: LIVING WITH ANXIETY AND PANIC DISORDERS

It is common for people to feel ashamed and be secretive about certain health conditions and people living with anxiety and panic disorders are no exemption. Even though there are group discussions where people share these experiences, for some people that is the limit of disclosure. What most of us do not realize is that we are not alone in this and apart from being with someone in it, there are those who have survived this phase and are now living happily. Anxiety disorders or panic disorders do not mean the end of the world; they are curable, but first proper diagnosis is necessary.

In this part, we see the stories of survivors of the different types of disorders; we also see how they overcame the situations.

3.0 YOU ARE NOT ALONE

> *"P.S. You're not going to die. Here's the white-hot truth: if you go bankrupt, you'll still be okay. If you lose the gig, the lover, the house, you'll still be okay. If you sing off-key, get beat by the competition, have your heart shattered, get fired... it's not going to kill you. Ask anyone who's been through it."*

Danielle LaPorte

These stories are not just for entertainment purposes. They serve to let people know that anxiety and panic are real; they are a way to show panic and anxiety sufferers that they can actually survive. If these people could do it, you can do it too.

Tammy:

Meet Tammy, a 29-year old graduate of Law. Tammy had everything going for her. A mom who loved her, a dad who was crazy about her, siblings who adored her and a boyfriend (Steve) who had been by her side since high school. Tammy graduated college just before her 21st birthday. Steve proposed to her on her 23rd birthday, and they got married six months later at the venue of her dreams, as if life itself was for Tammy alone; she had a set of twins (one boy and one girl) eleven months after her wedding.

Everything started with Tammy's pregnancy. She became easily irritated, suffered nausea, vomiting, insomnia, mood swings, hot and cold flashes, dizziness, abdominal cramping, headaches and the like. She went to see her gynecologist, who told her that they were normal with pregnancy and gave her some pills to reduce the symptoms.

After Tammy had her twins, the symptoms persisted and by this time, the anxiety had grown into an anxiety disorder. She paid a visit to a psychologist and after some interviews, she was diagnosed with anxiety and panic disorder. As an expectant mother, Tammy was worried that she would not make a great mother because her best friend, Lucy, was failing at motherhood. Her worry worsened when she discovered that she would have twins.

After childbirth, every time a kid cried (hers or another's) Tammy would suffer an attack. She would begin to suffer from shortness of breath, her mouth would go dry, she would experience an intense headache and the world would seem to spin; this would go on for about ten minutes and after she had calmed down, she would feel like she had just run a marathon.

You know what's funny? The very thing Tammy was worried about was what she became, and her excessive worry caused it. Panicking every time her children cried prevented her from giving them the necessary care they deserved; they cried and fell ill a lot. Tammy was usually never available. Tammy was having a miserable motherhood, sometimes she would tell herself that she was far worse than Lucy was, because Lucy may have been too busy for her kids, but she connected with them and always came to the rescue when she could. But in Tammy's case, she was never there, never.

The low point of her condition was when Yuri (Tammy's son) was four; while he was playing in a park, he slipped and was about to fall when he screamed. Tammy was the closest person to Yuri and would have caught her son if she reacted quickly but instead, she stood there thinking of all the things that could go wrong if Yuri fell. By the time she ran towards her son, he was on the grass but his ankle was sprained. Tammy blamed herself for this and never went to the park again.

On the brighter side, Steve tried to be there for Tammy as much as he could. He tried to calm her down during her attacks by using the magic words the psychologist had suggested. One day, while watching TV, the couple saw a documentary on "I would have died" about a woman who experienced a panic attack in a pool and nearly drowned. She told her story and how almost losing her life made her seek help immediately. She said she could not afford a shrink, so she sought a less expensive means of treatment.

The woman on the TV talked about dieting, yoga exercises, meditation and distraction. She encouraged people to embrace their fears and work out a means of survival. She said that she started doing these things eleven months before the show and it had been three months since her last attack; she was free!

It was at this point that it dawned on Tammy that, even though she was missing her doctor's appointments, there were other things she was doing which were worsening her condition too. The large chocolate bars she consumed daily, her constant coffee intake, the way she dwelt on the negative and fought her panic and anxiety attacks when they come. She made a conscious decision to fast from caffeine, tea, chocolate, fatty foods and high cholesterol foods, even though they were not causing weight gain. She started eating whole grains, including leafy vegetables, fish and poultry products, more dairy and lots of water. Tammy enrolled in a yoga class in her neighborhood and never missed a session; she practiced breathing exercises and read many books on positive thinking and relaxation. She decided that nothing would take her happiness away, nothing would deprive her the joy of witnessing her children's childhood and these were all she needed. In a few months, Tammy was fine!

Tammy now runs a center for black women suffering from panic and anxiety. She also proceeded to get a Diploma in Psychology and writes books on overcoming panic and anxiety. Tammy did all this after making a conscious decision to get better. It is not too late for you to make yours. Begin your healing process TODAY.

Kelvin:

I am Kelvin. Irrespective of my name, I come from Marfa, a small town in Texas. Yes, the same Marfa with the Prada-Marfa exhibit. I lived in Texas with my grandfather until I was eleven years old when I went off to an all-boys school in New York. I was excited to be going to the city even though my granddad and a host of others said that city life wasn't for me. When I arrived at the school, I immediately became close to Stan. Stan was two classes ahead of me but he was my roommate. He said he liked my freckles. Weird thing to like, I know.

Stan always watched my back, protected me from bullies and cared for me like a brother. He rolled well with the senior students for reasons unknown to me at the time. He changed my haircut to what he "preferred" and said it was cooler that way. Take note by the way, that the said hairstyle looked feminine, like one of Rihanna's haircuts. He made me tighten my trousers and the upper part of my shirts. He said my voice was too hoarse and made me drink some stuff to lighten my voice. Stan made me do a lot of strange stuff and I gradually started changing.

In my second year, I had a new roommate, Jerry. He was cool and didn't laugh at me for being so girly. He took me for who I was and we shared lots of stuff. After two months, I came back to my room and Jerry was gone – Stan was there, all smiley and shiny. I wasn't happy to see him, to be honest. My life was just beginning to take shape. Well, what can a boy do? I didn't know how he got there and I didn't know what would happen if I filed a report so – yeah, you guessed that right, I went with the flow.

Two weeks into having Stan as my roommate for the second time, I started feeling uncomfortable for no reason. I just felt something wasn't right about him. No, it wasn't the beginning of my attacks. My gut told me that all wasn't well and it was right! I was sleeping one cold evening when I felt something crawling up my lap; I wanted to slap it off but I didn't know the insect would bite so I brushed it off. Then it started to feel more like an animal than an insect so I jumped up. The animal put a cloth in my mouth, which muffled my scream. The strangest thing happened when the animal spoke and actually spoke in English. It said, "Keep still Kay, it's Stan." It still beats me why, but I did keep still.

Someone switched on the light. What touched me was no animal, it was Stan's fingers and he was standing over my bed with four boys whom I recognized from the soccer team. Then one of them, Eric, switched off the light and Stan switched on a lamp. They told me to keep quiet, or else they would pour candle wax on my manhood.

They took their turns having their way with me. It hurt; it hurt real bad, but it didn't hurt as much as the next eighteen years of my life. They kept doing this for a year, until a priest visited the school to see Simon, my tennis partner. I was with him when the priest came, so I started talking with the priest; he was easy to talk to; I told him everything that had been happening. I stayed back to practice more with Simon and by the time I got back to my room, Stan was gone and there was no roommate in my room.

Stan was gone, but something worse than Stan stayed back. My life became a nightmare. The life I thought was a wreck had worsened. I became a shadow of myself. I felt like the whole world now knew my story. I stopped going tennis practice, I avoided people a lot and I started misinterpreting any kind of interest a person of the same sex showed in me. I became socially detached and even asked for a new room.

I eventually changed schools, but this hardly solved anything. With time, I found myself keeping to my room (in the new school, there were no roommates). I studied hard and did well academically, but I never went out to my prizes. I took part in essay and poetry competitions, but I never attended the ceremonies to receive my awards. I was the valedictorian for my class, but I didn't deliver my valedictorian speech. I missed most of my glory moments because of this.

I still think it's a miracle that I made it through college. In college, I had just one friend, Sandra. She had interest in me for no reason. We were friends for a long time, even up to medical school. Sandra tried to give me a social life. I couldn't even join fraternities; I was always hanging out with the girls (if sitting in a tree and drinking lemonade while discussing pharmacology qualifies as hanging out). Sandra and her other friend (Vickie, quite promiscuous and raw) gave me all the support they could, Sandra most especially. I lived life through Sandra and I enjoyed her company more because she did not ask about my past. She just knew that I was terrified of male folk and reacted strangely around them, so she did her best to keep them away; she didn't even have a boyfriend!

One day, I told Sandra everything that happened with Stan. She felt so sorry for me and wished I had told her earlier. She found me a support group to join, which I did. In this group, we share our experiences and challenges. The group helped me begin to trust males again and I even got two male friends there. I was okay, just by talking to others and doing some pep talk myself.

Life was back to normal and everything was going smoothly; Sandra and I started seeing each other and our relationship was awesome! Everything changed when Sandra organized a candlelight dinner at home to surprise me. Immediately, when I saw the candlelight with the wax dripping, many negative images flashed through my mind. I analyzed everything and saw the possibility of Sandra forcing me to act against my will by using candle wax on me. I even thought of the best means of escape. I started sweating and trembling, my throat went dry and I could not swallow. I was having a severe headache and all I kept remembering were those nights at school and the possibility of a repeat. Sandra tried to get me to calm down but she came with a candlelight, which only worsened matters, my chest began to hurt terribly, I was so sure I was going to have a heart attack. She stayed away for some time and I eventually calmed down. Romantic dinner ruined.

That night, I had a nightmare of a repeat of that night but each dream, I saw Stan bringing the candle towards my balls. My room suddenly felt too small and I felt like it would suffocate me. I started having flashes of the rapes at random (both day and night) and my attacks worsened. One day, Sandra took me to see a friend who was a psychotherapist; I got help.

The psychotherapist started out a therapy routine with me; I spent many hours a month recounting the event many times until I became free with it, even made jokes out of it. I stayed in a room with many lit candles many times a week until I feared them no more. I used candle lights when I wanted to have a bath, get something from the fridge, etc. One day, I heard that Stan was in town. I searched until I found him, and I gave him a piece of my mind. I told him what his actions did to me. I told him that he ruined my life and had controlled it for so long and that all that was over because I was taking control again; I stormed out immediately after my speech.

Later that evening, Stan came over to my house to apologize. We had a candlelit dinner and I remember hyperventilating at some point, but my breathing exercises came through for me.

We moved out of that house to a bigger one. It was nine years into my marriage and I had never had sex with my wife. I didn't want to have a son that would face what I did; I wasn't even sure that I wouldn't be the one to do it to him. Sandra was a strong woman; despite the timelines and the pressure, she stayed by me.

In the tenth year of our marriage, we consummated it and I couldn't believe I had been a virgin all along. You cannot imagine the joy I felt knowing that she waited all these years. Well, by the time our son Jeremy was born, I realized that I hadn't had any attacks for the last year. I checked in with my doctor again and I was certified as clean and cured. That is the long and short of my story. It has inspired many people not to give up on their loved ones just because of one psychological issue or the other and it has encouraged sufferers of panic and anxiety to never give up on getting cured. I thought that I was damaged for life; I had condemned myself as unfit for society and had trust issues with people of the same sex. I was so sure that the rest of my life would slowly pass by and I would never be cured because I was convinced that my situation was the worst ever. However, I did it; you can do it too.

Janelle:

I come from a family of seven (now six); my mum died when I was seven. I'll tell you how she died because it is crucial to how this story goes. We were on a road trip to Tennessee. We were all singing along to Michael Jackson's "Thriller" that was playing on the car stereo; my Mum was a huge MJ fan. We were in the speed lane and the song had just ended when Mum suddenly started hyperventilating, she was trembling and then she began to cough incessantly; the worse part was that her eyes were closed. My siblings started screaming stuff like "What is wrong with you," "We're all gonna die," and "Do something, Mum." I noticed that in all this, my elder sister, 14 at the time, remained quiet. It was as if she didn't mind that the car was going off the road. I couldn't scream, my whole life flashed before my eyes, I was sure that it would be the end of us all. I thought of my Dad and hoped that he would live a good life without us. My eyes focused on my Mum and I saw her eyes open and saw the shock in her face just before the car hit a rock and we all surged forward. Long story short, my Mum died in that accident and I blamed her for her death and the motherless life I was living.

It was later, when I was twelve that Cheyenne (my elder sister) told me what was wrong with our mother, and why she acted and subsequently died the way she did. She said that Mum was working three jobs and slept three to four hours a night; she was always drinking coffee and took Valium to help her sleep. Cheyenne had walked in on Mum and Dad talking and Dad was telling Mum to quit one of her jobs, that the family could do without a few hundred dollars extra, and that he was getting a big promotion, but Mum would not hear of it. Dad reminded her that a psychological disorder ran in her family and she was only increasing its likelihood by stressing herself out much and consuming so much caffeine (he didn't know about the Valium). Mum was upset and said that he was insulting her because she was black; she accused him of being racist and condemned him for reminding her of her family history. Cheyenne said that four days later, Mum had an attack similar to the one she had in the car and that day, she spilled hot coffee on herself. Cheyenne cleaned her up and applied some ointment. Mum told her that everything was fine. It didn't happen again until the accident that claimed her life (two months later).

I later understood (at age fifteen) that my grandma was suffering from depression and anxiety disorder and what my mum had experienced was panic. I immediately searched the conditions and realized that they were hereditary. I started anticipating an attack; I kept away from stuff like driving, cheerleading, crossing busy roads without stress, and any other thing that could put me in a position of danger if an attack came. I even started taking Prozac and Propranolol to kill the condition before it manifested. Later, I started staying away from people. I became ashamed (of a condition I wasn't sure I suffered from).

By age 20, I had never had a boyfriend because I wasn't sure how long I had to live, so I didn't want to break his heart by dying on him (probably during sex). I was sure that an attack was imminent and that I would die from it. I even kept away from exercising so that my heartrate wouldn't increase and the attack would seize that opportunity to manifest. I was so scared of getting a panic attack that I increased my Propranolol intake and added Tofranil to the mix.

I was always at home, except when I needed groceries (which I only purchased at night). I was dizzy most of the time, my stomach ached a lot, I couldn't keep down anything I ate and I had difficulty remembering stuff. At one point, I quit school. Cheyenne came over to Atlanta to see me; I was a mess. I was hallucinating and talking gibberish, I had swollen feet and lips, she was sure I was hurting myself. She took me to a small hospital where a doctor recommended psychiatric care.

I spent nine months receiving psychiatric care and even though I passed through a lot there, those days turned my life around for good. Things were getting better until one day, when we were watching TV, I saw a movie about a woman who killed all her kids in an accident because she was high on cocaine. I froze immediately, my hands were sweaty, I couldn't breathe, and I kept seeing flashes of the accident and most of my past life flashed before me. I was shaking vigorously and the room started spinning. I could hear voices, but they were faint. I saw white flashes and then darkness (I passed out). After that incident, I started keeping to myself again, and I stopped watching television.

Well, long story short, Cheyenne forced me to see a doctor and I was diagnosed with acute agoraphobia and panic disorder. The doctor recommended many things, including taking a holiday. I went to Hawaii and the first week there was agonizing for me because I had to keep running into people. My doctor kept checking on me, we had video calls, he checked my diet, my sleep hours, my social life and a host of other things. He also recommended that I drive around aimlessly for one hour a day, that was when we realized that I didn't know the first thing about driving (at age 28). I started driving lessons, passed the test and got a license.

My doctor's name is Dr. Morris; he is my husband now and we have two beautiful daughters together. It's been four years since and I haven't had any attacks or issues with psychological disorders. Not only am I cured, I am healed because I feel like it will never happen again. Therefore, I want you to know that everyone can live a disorder-free life; it begins with talking to someone about it so that you can get help.

Most of the things that helped me are:

- Social Inclusion and Exposure – This was the most challenging part for me and I may not recommend this to any agoraphobic patient because it is a daunting task, but it did a lot for me. It was my big step and I think you should try it too (Okay, there, I recommended it).
- Meditation – I did a lot of meditation and the calm it brought is the best. It penetrates every part of your daily activity, giving you comfort, balance and reassurance. In my daughter's words, "Meditation is BAE."
- Breathing Exercises: I learnt how to take slow breaths through the diaphragm.
- I read many self-help books and acted on the advice therein to boost my self-esteem and improve my self-confidence.
- Learning how to feel my muscular tension and how to release it. I learnt this through meditation too and it helps a great deal.
- Appreciating that panic was just the fight or flight response and that I wasn't having a heart attack or dying

- Exercises: I gained a lot of weight as a side effect of the drugs I was taking, but I also lost a big chunk of it. I took up long distance jogging and other aerobic exercises.
- Nutrition: I ate whole grains, especially brown rice and lentils, green vegetables, many salmon diets and some Vitamin supplements.
- Knowing that I deserved a break: I rested when I felt tired, never forced work on myself and didn't agree to any request that would stress me out. I avoided short deadlines and pressure.

These stories aren't just for entertainment purposes. Moreover, they are a poor representation of the number of people who have been through different types of anxiety disorders, including panic disorders, and were treated even after they gave up on life. As you can see from these few stories, the cure did not happen immediately, neither did it come to meet them while they were sulking somewhere and wallowing in self-pity or hate for the world. They made conscious efforts to get help, like talking to someone about it. It is okay to be shy or ashamed of your situation, but that shouldn't last more than a day or two. The only reason why you're not getting help is you. Girl, you must stand up and make the necessary changes. Do what you must do to the live the happy life you deserve. Are you confused about what to do? You will find the answers in the subsequent pages. Read on.

3.1 EFFECTS OF ANXIETY AND PANIC DISORDERS

Anxiety has both long-term and short-term effects on the patient and these effects may vary from person to person depending on the level and type of anxiety disorder they are suffering from. In this section, we shall briefly look at the general effects of anxiety.

1. SHORT-TERM EFFECTS

- Difficulty Swallowing: During an anxiety or panic attack, a person may notice that they are unable to swallow; they try but nothing is going down, this could make them more anxious.

- Dizziness: This creates a false impression that the patient's environment is spinning and he or she is about to fall, this may either cause them to freeze or scream. In anxiety, it could cause panic but in panic, it will worsen.
- Dry Mouth: It is not wrong to assume that the salivary glands stop functioning during an Anxiety or Panic attack. The mouth suddenly becomes dry; this contributes to difficulty swallowing and may lead to choking.
- Rapid heartbeat: Every abnormal hormonal or bodily function affects heart rate in one way or the other. During an anxiety attack or a panic attack, the body goes into survival mode because of the amount of negative messages that are sent to the brain and the increased breaths taken by the patient that leads to an increased heart rate.
- Rapid Breathing and Shortness of Breath: Hyperventilation occurs because of increased heart rate.
- Fatigue: After an attack, a person is drained and tired just as it happens with panic attacks. This is why rest is recommended, especially if the anxiety was caused by stress.
- Headaches: This doesn't happen with everyone, but most people experience severe headache before and after an anxiety or panic attack.
- Inability to concentrate: The entire focus of the patient is either on how to survive the attack or the cause of the attack, so it becomes difficult to focus on other activities, as important as they may be.
- Irritability: This is common with both disorders.
- Muscle Aches: It happens because of the stress of the attack.
- Muscle Tension: This is due to the fatigue that comes with anxiety or panic attacks.

- Nausea: Irritability and fear have a way of creating a feeling of vomiting and for persons who are scared of vomiting, this could worsen their anxiety.
- Sweating: When a person is under any form of attack, physical, psychological or emotional, perspiration may occur.
- Trembling and Twitching: It is an indication of fear and happens during and after panic or anxiety attacks.

2. LONG-TERM EFFECTS

People with prolonged, untreated cases of anxiety disorder are more likely to suffer these effects. They come about because of a constant experience of the short-term effects that cause strain on some major body parts, thus reducing their potency.

- **Insomnia:** Insomnia often goes hand-in-hand with anxiety. Insomnia can cause anxiety; in the same vein, anxiety can lead to insomnia. Insomnia is usually one of the first symptoms of anxiety.
- **Increased risk of stroke:** The continuous release of "flight or fight hormones" increases risks to the heart. Research suggests that middle-aged men experiencing symptoms of psychological distress are more than 3 times as likely to have a fatal stroke.
- **Early memory decline:** Anxiety may cause long-term damage to hippocampus cells, which have negative effects on memory and learning. Consequently, anxiety can bring about early memory decline, especially in elderly patients or sufferers.
- **Detrimental impact of emotional distraction:** As discussed above, anxiety can induce a lack of concentration, which may mean low academic performance or poor attitude to work as well as an inability to maintain relationships with their family, friends, colleagues and other loved ones.

3. POSITIVE EFFECTS

It probably sounds strange but there are positive effects to a condition as painful as panic and anxiety Disorders. Some of these benefits are as discussed below:

- Warning: According to Dr. Jeremy Coplan who conducted a study on Anxiety patients, *"While excessive worry is generally seen as a negative trait and high intelligence as a positive one, worry may cause our species to avoid dangerous situations, regardless of how remote a possibility they may be."* Anxiety and panic sufferers get a forewarning of impending danger and this could act to save the patient's life or properties as well as the lives of those around the patient. They avoid situations and places that pose potential danger and encourage their close ones to do it, thus they avoid dark alleys, drugs and many other places where they could suffer some damage.

- Preparation and Success: Anxiety over say a test makes the anxious person prepare far harder than their contemporaries and so some of them are seen excelling in school and making high grades.

- Preservation of Life: On one hand, one could interpret it as cowardice but on the other hand, an anxious person is less likely to involve his or herself in situations that cause a feeling of fear in them, so they avoid these situations. Most of these situations are dangerous ones and you see them living longer because they escape some negative occurrences, which could have cost them their lives. It is safe to say that they protect and continue the human race.

- Fun and Relaxation: Generally, stress causes increased levels of brain chemicals known as dopamine, endorphins, and serotonin, which help calm people down during uncomfortable moments. Competition, whether among political rivals, athletes, students or coworkers, can produce anxiety, but this anxiety only serves to help them make strategic plans or work towards goals to achieve successful results. In most cases, the competition becomes a fun affair.

- Increased Functionality: During anxiety attacks, a surge of adrenaline is released which immediately puts the mind in alert mode and increases energy levels in the body. In the face of real danger, we find that anxious people run at a speed they didn't know they could and move very heavy objects to save not just themselves but people around them. They become the heroes of the day.

4. THE SUICIDAL EFFECT

Both depression and anxiety carry a high risk of suicide. More than 90 percent of those who die by suicide have a diagnosable illness such as clinical depression, and often in combination with anxiety or substance use disorders and other treatable mental disorders."

Mark Pollack, MD, ADAA; Past President and Grainger Professor and Chairman, Department of Psychiatry at Rush University Medical Center (emphasis mine)

Suicide is one of the top leading causes of death, especially in the United States, and research has revealed that most suicide attempters are diagnosed with anxiety disorders or panic disorders either before or after the suicide attempt. Some of the people who suffer anxiety and panic attacks spend their free time thinking of how terrible life is because of their condition. They construct the means to cover up the problem and protect themselves from public shame. At a point, the scheming and games stop working and the secret is out. While some are lucky to have people who understand the situation and offer support, others are unfortunate to be surrounded by impatient and ignorant people who are either oblivious of what is happening or have no interest in offering assistance. Although the people in the former category consider suicide, the majority of those in the latter category do not just consider it, they commit suicide. This is the suicidal effect of Anxiety and it is common with panic attack sufferers.

Close and loved ones of panic and anxiety sufferers as well as society can prevent suicide if they take note of certain pointers to this act and take adequate action. According to the Anxiety and Depression Association of America (ADAA), to prevent others from committing suicide, people should look out for the following:

Talk
If a person talks about:
- Being a burden to others
- Feeling trapped
- Experiencing unbearable pain
- Having no reason to live
- Killing themselves

Behavior
Specific things to look out for include:
- Increased use of alcohol or drugs
- Looking for a way to kill themselves, such as searching online for materials or means
- Acting recklessly
- Withdrawing from activities
- Isolating from family and friends
- Sleeping too much or too little
- Visiting or calling people to say goodbye
- Giving away prized possessions
- Aggression

Mood
People who are considering suicide often display one or more of the following moods:

- Depression
- Loss of interest
- Rage
- Irritability
- Humiliation
- Anxiety

When you notice any of these, get help immediately. If you try talking them out of it directly and by yourself, they might decide to do it at an earlier time than they had planned to. It is thus wise to involve either a specialist, a loved and respected person or a calm adult (where no specialist is available). When you have successfully dissuaded the person, let him or her get help immediately. Where you cannot reach any of these persons, start by telling them all the good things about life, how much you love them, how it would break your heart to lose them and how special they are. Secure the area by keeping lethal things like drugs, knives, guns and sharp objects at bay. If you are on the first floor or a higher floor, you may need to lock the windows.

Keep them talking, let them pour out their heart to you and make sure you show that you are interested in what they are saying. Observe them for any strange reactions or movements; they may have already hurt themselves before you got there. You could also connect them to the people they cherish and respect the most for them to talk to about any subject matter. Find out the reason for their suicidal plans and try to rebut them calmly.

You may succeed in dissuading them that day, but it doesn't end there. Get them professional care immediately and try to follow up with them by staying in touch. Assure them that they aren't alone and always remind them of how special and important they are to you and the world. It is also wise to have emergency numbers on speed dial.

If the suicide attempt is already in progress, that is, if they already took an overdose, shot themselves, jumped from a high place or did anything deadly, try not to panic. Administer the necessary First Aid treatment while calling for help (all kinds of positive help; professional, emergency, local). DO EVERYTHING POSSIBLE to save their lives. They may hate you a bit but this will change and they may be eternally grateful when they realize the value of what you did for them.

The rule of thumb is to try hard not to panic when you meet a person who is attempting or has attempted suicide. Panic affects rational thinking and wastes time that you could spend saving a life.

PART 4: PREVENTION, CARE AND REMEDIES

4.0 PREVENTION OF ANXIETY DISORDERS

The activities and mechanisms to facilitate living an anxiety disorder-free life are generally easy, but could be difficult for some people (especially those who have grown dependent or addicted to the medicines). This is not a fool-proof method of prevention, but it goes a long way to help. To prevent anxiety disorders by keeping anxious emotions at bay:

- Maintain a healthy diet by including whole grains, fish (fatty fish) and poultry, dairy products, fruits and vegetables in your meals.
- Reduce the intake of caffeine, cola, chocolate and tea.
- Avoid alcohol.
- Maintain a regular sleep pattern.
- Before using herbal remedies or OTCDs, (Over-the-Counter Drugs) check with a doctor or pharmacist to make sure they do not contain chemicals that may worsen anxiety.
- Stay away from cannabis sativa and other recreational drugs.
- If you are already addicted to hard substances like cocaine, cannabis, etc. seek help immediately.

4.1 PREVENTION OF PANIC DISORDERS

Panic attacks are stressful, they leave the victim distressed and exhausted when they subside. It isn't just energy draining, it is time-wasting too, because apart from the time spent waiting for the attack to subside, more time is spent waiting for the victim to recover properly. As stated in an earlier part of this book, panic disorders are diagnosed from repeated sudden panic attacks; therefore, preventing a panic attack is invariably preventing panic disorder.

To prevent panic disorders before they begin, follow these tips:

- **Adapt to Triggers:** One of the ways to do this is desensitization. While it is best to do this in the presence of a trained expert or a therapist, desensitization is the act of conforming to your triggers until they no longer cause anxiety. For instance, if you find that dizziness tends to trigger your panic attacks, try to get used to dizziness by deliberately inducing it (maybe by spinning around in a chair or a circle). You can hyperventilate on purpose; get your heartbeat up by running in place - there are varieties of strategies you can use to get used to each physical trigger of your panic attacks so that they cause less fear when they happen, just get creative.

- **Control Your Breathing:** It is more effective if you start by learning to control your breath anytime you hyperventilate. The key to breath control is taking slow deliberate breaths and fighting the urge to breathe too quickly or fully.

  Try to take 14 to 15 seconds for one full breath in total. Use 5 seconds to breath in, hold your breath for 2 or 3 seconds, and then breathe slowly out for the remaining 7 seconds. Doing this whenever there is an imminent panic attack may not totally stop the attack but it can mitigate its severity.

- **Visit the Doctor:** Health issues rarely induce panic attacks but a regular visit to a doctor is an important part of getting the reassurance needed to proceed with panic attack treatments. Ruling out health problems as causes will make it easier for you to manage the panic attacks.

  However, hearing from a doctor does not miraculously stop the pessimistic voice in your head that makes you worry about your health.

- **Start Talking About It:** It is common for sufferers of panic attacks to feel embarrassed about the attacks and try to fight them when they occur (which worsens it). When you are out in public - or even sitting alone in a park and you start having that feeling that something isn't right, the reflexive action is to try to push it away and fix it yourself. You need to get outside your own thoughts as much as you can. Therefore, be fine with talking to those around you about it or calling someone you trust to let them know how you're feeling.

- **Exercise:** This is ironic because exercise can cause panic attacks in some people because of how their minds interpret heart rate and fatigue. However, it doubles as a powerful anxiety reduction tool; it provides a similar mental health benefit to many anxiety medications. Discuss exercising more with your doctor, because while it is a big addition to any anxiety reduction plan, doing it wrongly could worsen the situation.

- **Maintain a Healthy Lifestyle:** Living healthy is not just important for avoiding panic attacks but for staying healthy generally. Diet plays a big part here, and you must ensure that you are getting sufficient vitamins since vitamin deficiencies can cause some discomforts that may trigger panic attacks. Sleep is perhaps the most important aspect of healthy living because sleep debt causes a legion of symptoms that tend to trigger panic attacks, like lack of focus, headaches, stiff muscles, and weakness.

- **Allow the Attack:** Allowing an attack is probably one of the toughest things you can do but it is also one of the most important things. You need to be fine with having panic attacks. That means if you discover that you get panic attacks when you go to a particular place, the park for instance, then you still have to go to that park when you need to. Do not pass on the opportunity to go there just because you get panic attacks there. Get comfortable with the idea that a panic attack could happen and brace for it. If or when it occurs, wait it out, and then go on with your day's activities as planned. Do not give a panic attack the right to ruin your plans.

- **Practice Relaxation Techniques:** This starts with as little as relaxing your facial muscles to as big as incorporating yoga and meditation into your daily routine. When your facial muscles are relaxed, it is an indication that there is little or nothing to worry about and this affects how certain hormones act in you to either relieve stress or enhance it.

It is no news that yoga and meditation relax the mind, free it of negativity and enhance inner peace. Imagine a life where you had no time for worries. We are not asking you to pretend that you don't have issues or challenges, we're saying that you should realize that worrying over them doesn't change the fact that they exist, so why beat yourself up about it?

- **Find Practical Solutions:** While worrying and keeping vigil over life's issues does nothing to improve them, do you know what does? Seeking a solution. Are you worried that you may never have kids? Visit your doctor and find out. If it is true then immediately start discussing your options (surrogacy, adoption, etc.) because dwelling on the problem of infertility never caused fertility. Is it the bills? Instead of thinking of how overwhelming they are and how little your income is, why not start by paying off the ones you can and see what progress you make? There is no problem without a solution and even if the solution is unknown, you shouldn't kill yourself over it.

- **Be Content; Stop Looking for Fairytale Endings:** Sometimes, we expect too much from life and from people; we try to ignore the possibility of failure and so when it comes, it tears us down and crushes our self-esteem. Some of us allow the timelines set by society to weigh us down and we become anxious about meeting them. Graduating college at 21 and getting married before 25 is not the standard rule for living. Girl, you have your whole life ahead of you and if something prevents you from graduating, even at 26, it doesn't mean that you are a failure. The funny thing is that most people who worry about these may be successful in other spheres of their lives. For instance, a woman who is a CEO at 27 is worried that she wasn't able to settle down with a man at 25; another woman who finished college at 21, got married at 23 and then had a kid immediately is disturbed that at 28 she doesn't have another kid coming.

We must understand that in life, we cannot have it all and so we must learn to be grateful for the little things we have and accept the things we cannot change, because no matter how bad you think your life is, there is someone out there who is doing a lot worse than you are.

4.2 CARE FOR THOSE LIVING WITH ANXIETY AND PANIC DISORDERS

For sufferers of panic and anxiety, especially those with friends and family members who do not understand what they go through, it is reassuring and relaxing to know that the people around them won't just be there when they get these attacks, but will be there for them always. It is for this reason that it is important to have certain tips at your disposal so that rather than run helter-skelter when a close one is attacked with panic or anxiety, you can make yourself useful in calming them down and saving the situation. The following tips come in handy during a panic or anxiety attack:

- Do not freak out when they start; be calm.
- Locate their medication if it is available and ensure that they take it.
- Gently suggest things you both (say 'we' instead of 'you') can do to distract the patient from the anxiety or panic causing thought or event.
- Acknowledge their distress and offer yourself as available to do anything that could help.
- Encourage them to take short, deep breaths.
- Keep breathing with them.
- If the panic is dissociative, remind them that it has happened before and they survived, so the current one shall pass too.

- Assure them that they aren't alone, that you are there with them.
- Give them a long, warm (not suffocating) hug and tell them that everything will be fine.
- Calmly recount their beautiful or happy memories to them and tell them about their achievements, let them know how proud this makes you of them.
- Remind them that it is better to let the attack pass than fight it, as the former is worse than the latter.
- If it is beyond your control, call a specialist ASAP!

No matter how freaked out you get when you witness a panic or anxiety attack, do not use the following words or their synonyms:

- "Suck it Up"
  It makes them feel that they are bothering you; they become more embarrassed so the attack only worsens. It makes them feel that they're too weak to handle their problems.
- "Stop It"
  If a panic or anxiety attack were something that a person could just stop, you probably wouldn't witness it. It is uncontrollable and involuntary, they don't enjoy it, but they cannot just stop it.
- "Don't worry about it" or "Don't think about it"
  This may seem strange, but dishing out this order doesn't solve anything. It has a paradoxical effect, especially as the human brain usually highlights subject matter it is told not to worry about or think of.
- "Can't you just calm down?"
  If they could, they would not need you to tell them to do so. As stated earlier, there is no abrupt solution to anxiety or panic attacks, so suggesting it - whether calmly or harshly - has a counterproductive effect.
- "You're fine."
  "You'll be fine" is more like it. Psychologists equate the level of anxiety during an attack to the feeling you

get when a gun is pointed to your head. Therefore, they are not fine, reassurance is what they need, not lies.

Lashing out at sufferers of panic or anxiety attacks could damage your relationship with them; they begin to feel that they are not safe around you and so cannot trust you, especially not with their lives when they are in danger.

4.3 REMEDIES FOR ANXIETY AND PANIC DISORDERS: A STEP-BY-STEP GUIDE

- NATURAL REMEDIES

Most anxiety and panic patients do not use medication because they are prone to becoming dependent on the drugs, which is why therapy and natural remedies are highly recommended. There are certain natural foods, herbs or drinks, as well as plants, that could provide a temporary solution to anxiety.

Chamomile Tea: Chamomile tea belongs to the *Asteraceae/Compositae* family and is represented by two common varieties: German Chamomile (*Chamomilla recutita*) and Roman Chamomile (*Chamaemelum nobile*). In its dried form, chamomile flowers contain terpenoids and flavonoids that contribute to its medicinal properties. The compound (Matricaria recutita) in chamomile tea has a calming effect on an anxious mind because it binds to the same brain receptors as Valium does.

A study in Hamburg, Germany revealed that when taken with other extracts from plants within the Compositae family, German Chamomile might cause allergic reactions in certain people. However, the FDA has enlisted it in the GRAS (Generally Recognized as Safe) list. Safety in young children, pregnant women or nursing mothers, or persons with liver or kidney disease has not been established, although there have not been any credible reports of toxicity caused by this common beverage tea.

At the University of Pennsylvania Medical Center in Philadelphia, a study revealed that patients who consumed chamomile tea for eight weeks saw a significant reduction in anxiety symptoms versus patients who received a placebo.

The common dosage for chamomile extract is 220-milligram capsules but one should confer with their doctor before using this drug.

Lemon Balm (*Melissa officinalis*): Since the middle ages, lemon balm has served as a mild sedative to reduce stress and anxiety and aid sleep. Eighteen healthy volunteers took part in a study showing that a group who took 600mg of lemon extract was calmer than the group that consumed a placebo.

While it is effective, research reveals that an excessive intake of this substance can lead to more anxiety, thus it is advisable to begin with small doses. The herb is commercially available as capsules, tea and tincture and is safe to combine with other herbs like chamomile, hops and valerian.

Griffonia simplicifolia (5-HTP): The African shrub is the most important commercial source of 5-hydroxytryptophan (HTP), an amino acid that the body turns into serotonin. The seeds contain up to 20 percent 5-HTP by weight and in African folk medicine, they are used to cure many ailments.
Presently, *Griffonia simplicifolia* is used to relieve anxiety and boost moods because the 5-HTP in it works like SSRIs such as Prozac and Zoloft.
Like these drugs, 5-HTP works by increasing serotonin levels within the brain, thus causing a reduction in anxiety, depression, insomnia, and other neurological issues.

The recommended dosage for this shrub is 50 milligrams one to three times daily.

Valerian *(Valeriana officinalis)*: This herb has a double effect of reducing anxiety and inducing sleep so it is advisable to take it in the evening. It also works to reduce stress and panic attacks by enhancing GABA signaling. Valerian is good because it enhances sleep at night and daytime alertness. If taken properly, it can solve anxiety and panic issues.

The useful components of the Valerian plant are the roots, horizontal stem and in some cases, the leaves. Because of its offensive smell, most people would rather consume it as a capsule or tincture than as a tea, but it is available in all three forms. It is safe to combine it with other herbs like hops, lemon balm and chamomile, this mixture provides better efficacy. The proper dosage is 300 to 900 mg a day.

Despite its abilities, Valerian has side effects but these side effects are rare. The reactions include:Swelling of the facial features (lips, tongue, and the face)

- Anaphylactic shock
- Drowsiness
- Shortness of breath
- Uneasiness
- Constipation
- Dry mouth
- Diarrhea
- Autoimmune conditions (Psoriasis, Rheumatoid arthritis)
- High cholesterol levels

To reduce the effects, take Valerian as prescribed by your doctor, pharmacist or herbal practitioner. Stomach conditions (constipation and diarrhea) are common with Valerian in its capsule or pill form; taking it as tea or tincture can solve this for some people. Also, take it short-term, over a three to six month period. While high doses can induce sleep, it is not advisable to take it for a period beyond one month.

Valerian is not suitable for use by:

- Pregnant women
- Nursing mothers
- Persons addicted to drugs or alcohol
- Children (unless as recommended by a pediatrician)
- People who are on other medications like Tramadol, Cymbalta, Benadryl, trazodone, and Xanax, and high doses of other herbs like St. John's Wort.

Hops *(Humulus Lupulus)*: You guessed right, it's contained in beer but this is not to suggest that consuming beer will have the same effects as taking hops in its independent form. Many specialists know hops fruits for their anxiolytic components.

The sedative compound in this herb is a volatile oil, so it is contained in extracts and tinctures and in hops pillows as aromatherapy. Apart from its volatile component, hops is quite bitter and therefore people consume it with chamomile or Valerian.

The bitter resins in hops trigger GABA, which blocks neurotransmitters that trigger anxiety, irritability, nervousness and panic.

Ginkgo Biloba: Although known for brain stimulation and preventing memory loss, ginkgo can also reduce anxiety in humans. Scientists suggest that the flavonoids and terpenoids found in ginkgo extract reduce corticosterone levels, which could lessen anxiety and improve brain function by aiding memory retention.

Ginkgo is available in capsules, extracts and tinctures. A typical dose of the drug is between 120 and 360 mgs each day but this is dependent on the condition treated and thus patients should consume according to prescription. It is dangerous to combine ginkgo biloba with SSRIs, such as Zoloft and Lexapro.

There are no known serious side effects of taking ginkgo but an overdose is very dangerous and may cause hyperactivity.

Passionflower: No, this is no love potion. In fact, it is a sedative. It should not accompany any other sedative herb or prescription sedative. It works with GABA to reduce anxiety.

The recommended doses are:
- 1 teaspoon of the dried leaves for tea
- 10 to 20 drops of the extract thrice a day or
- Up to 45 drops in a diluted tincture form.

Passionflower also works well when combined with lemon balm and other herbs. One should not take Passionflower beyond a period of one month to avoid negative side effects.

Cherimoya (*Annona cherimolia*): This tropical fruit tree is also called graviola, custard apple, or soursop, but it is not just a fruit. Research shows that the alkaloids in the leaves and aerial portions of *Annona cherimolia* and other species in the same genus had antidepressant-like effects. The alkaloids interact with serotonin receptors, modulate dopamine transmission and improve the ratio rates of both neurotransmitters.

Evidence also exists that cherimoya alkaloids treat anxiety because they help regulate GABA, which blocks anxiety-producing nerve signals in the body.

One can brew powdered leaves into a calmative tea and drink it up to three times a day. The recommended dosage is 1 teaspoon of the powder for every 6 ounces of water.

Lavender (*Lavandula hybrida*): The lavender plant has a sweet, intoxicating (but safe) smell that could be an "emotional" inflammatory. A Greek study indicated that anxiety patients tend to feel calmer when they find themselves in rooms scented with lavender oil. A study conducted on students in Florida showed that students who inhaled lavender before an exam experienced a decrease in their anxiety but some complained that they felt "fuzzy" during the exam.

It was revealed in a German study that a pill made from lavender caused an effective reduction in anxiety as would lorazepam (brand name: Ativan), (which is an anti-anxiety medication in the same class as Valium) when administered to people with GAD (General Anxiety Disorder).

The proper dosage is 80 to 100 mgs a day but this is subject to your doctor's prescription.

L-theanine (Green Tea): Rich in amino acids, a good consumption of this is effective for regulating heartrate, blood pressure and reducing anxiety. 200mg of L-theanine can cause immediate relief but this would require consuming 5 to 20 cups of green tea.

Other useful herbs and plants include St. John's Wort, Kava kava (note that this medicine is very dangerous as its use can cause liver problems), Flaxseed oil, Schisandra (Wu-wei-zi), Eucalyptus, Licorice root, Holy basil, Skullcap, etc.

Ashwagandha (*Withania somnifera*): This Indian herb is regarded as the ginseng of Ayurvedic medicine. Both the root and the berries of his herb have many medicinal applications that researchers are still exploring. So far, Ashwagandha qualifies as an effective Adaptogen that helps the body deal with everyday stressors.

At the end of a 60-day study published in a 2012 edition of the Indian Journal of Psychological Medicine, patients with chronic stress who consumed 300 mgs of Ashwagandha had lower cortisol levels, felt more relaxed and were more stress resistant than those who were given a placebo.

Most studies that compared the effects of *Withania somnifera* to benzodiazepines show that the herb reduced anxiety levels by 56 percent.

The suggested daily dosage is between 300 and 500 milligrams.

Note:

These herbs and fruits are a source of hope to anxiety and panic sufferers who may not be able to afford professional help, either due to finance or other inhibitions. They function like Benzodiazepines to increase GABA levels while others act like SSRIs to increase neurotransmitters that boost relaxation and happiness.

While this may look like an easy miracle for anxiety and panic patients, the consequences of abusing these herbs are grave. Therefore, for safety and health purposes only, use these herbs to treat your condition after your doctor has ascertained the safety of using it. DO NOT consume any of the sedatives mentioned above with other sedatives unless otherwise directed by a doctor or pharmacist. Inform your doctor on the various supplements you are consuming or have consumed. Also, REMEMBER that these are just temporary reliefs and should not be relied upon for total cure of anxiety or panic.

- MEDICATIONS, DOSAGES AND SIDE EFFECTS

There are many medicines available for treating panic and anxiety disorders and most of them have side effects. In this section, we shall look at the drugs, their dosages and side effects.

a. PROPRANOLOL

It is a generic drug. In other words, it does not have any brand name and this makes it cheaper than other drugs in the *Beta Blockers* class of drugs to which it belongs. It comes in four basic forms, injectable, oral tablet, extended-release oral capsule, and oral liquid solution.

Its mode of operation in affecting treatment is still unknown. It is a non-selective Beta-receptive drug so it works equally on all organs - heart, kidney, lungs and liver. In its oral form, Propranolol regularizes the heart rate thus solving one anxiety and panic symptom. The drug also serves to treat tremors, atrial fibrillation and prevent migraines.

SIDE EFFECTS AND WARNINGS

- **Drowsiness:** The drug has some sedative contents that could cause drowsiness so until you have confirmed how this drug affects you, it is wise to avoid engaging in activities like controlling heavy machinery, driving, piloting or any other act that requires alertness.
- **Asthma:** Propranolol is bad for all asthma patients. It is important to verify that one is not an asthma patient before administering the drug or taking it because it could worsen asthma.
- **Low Blood Sugar:** Apart from causing low blood sugar (Hypoglycemia), Propranolol can conceal some symptoms of low blood sugar by normalizing a high heart rate and preventing shaking or sweating. Persons with diabetes should be cautious while taking this drug, especially if they are taking insulin or other drugs that reduce blood sugar. Infants, children and adults who do not suffer from diabetes could get hypoglycemic by consuming this drug, especially if the adults have just concluded strenuous exercises or have kidney issues.
- **When to stop treatment:** It is common for people to quit taking certain medication (without completing the dosage) when the symptoms they are treating seem to have stopped. For propranolol, it is wrong to decide to stop taking the medication on one's own. Quitting this medication should only come with doctor's recommendation. The effects of sudden stoppage vary among persons but include an increase in blood pressure, worsened chest pain, irregular heart rate, and the like, but a physician would know how to lower the dosages to prevent these effects.
- **Other Side Effects:** Decreased heart rate, hair loss, dry eyes, tiredness, dizziness, diarrhea, dry or peeling

skin, vomiting, skin rash, changes in blood sugar, itching, nightmares, insomnia, hallucinations, cold hands or feet, sudden weight gain, facial swelling, swelling of ankles and legs, etc.

DOSAGES

There are special dosage considerations for people who have kidney or liver problems, so doctors should use caution when prescribing Propranolol for them.

Take as Directed by the Doctor: If a person doesn't take Propranolol as directed by the physician, symptoms could worsen or even grow into a more grievous health condition. The effects of abusing the drug are:

Failure to take it at all: Your condition will get worse and you may be at risk of serious heart problems, such as heart attack or stroke.

Taking too much: If you think you have taken too much of this drug, call your doctor or local poison control center. If your symptoms are severe, call 911 or go to the nearest emergency room right away.

Skipping or missing doses: Skipping a dose may worsen the patient's condition. If one skips or misses a dose, take it as soon as you remember. If it is close to the time of your next dose, only take one dose at that time. Taking a double-dose as a way to make up for the missed dose can cause dangerous effects and is best avoided.

The drug is working if the symptoms are improving. For example, the blood pressure and heart rate of the consumer should be lower, or the person should begin to experience less chest pain, tremors or shaking.

Important Considerations When Taking Propranolol

If the doctor prescribes propranolol for a person, they should keep the following considerations in mind:

General Considerations

- Take the drug before meals and at bedtime.
- The tablet can either be cut or crushed before consumption

Storage

- Tablets should be stored between 59°F to 86°F (15°C to 30°C).
- Protect the drug from light.
- Do not store this medication in damp or moist areas, like drug cabinets in bathrooms.

Refills

If a single prescription is insufficient for a complete dosage, the doctor will write the number of refills authorized while prescribing the medicine so that a new prescription will be unnecessary to get a refill.

Travel

If the need arises to travel while taking this medication, then:

- Always take the drug along. If the means of transport is flight, never put it into a checked bag; keep it in the hand luggage. Do not be perturbed about airport x-ray machines because they cannot harm the medication.
- You may need to show airport staff the pharmacy label for your medication. Always carry the original prescription-labeled container with you.
- Be sure to avoid leaving the medicine in a car's glove compartment or in the car at all when the weather is very hot or very cold.

Self-management

While taking propranolol, one needs need to monitor their:

- Heart rate
- Blood pressure
- Blood sugar (for diabetic patients)

Clinical Monitoring

After prescription doctor will conduct periodic blood tests on his patient to check the following:

- Liver function
- Kidney function
- Electrolyte levels
- Heart function

Availability

Propranolol is not a drug that is readily available in every pharmacy so it is important to call ahead while filling out the prescription to be sure that it is available.

Alternatives to Propranolol

Some pharmacists usually suggest alternatives to drugs, especially when they do not have them, even though these alternatives may work, this is not the case with Propranolol because while there may be drugs to handle the situation, some might be better than others. If Propranolol is unavailable, talking to the doctor about other options is the best call to make.

b. ALPRAZOLAM

It is a Benzodiazepine. It affects the chemicals that may be unbalanced in the brains of anxiety patients. Another drug in this class is Lorazepam.

Side Effects and Warning

The common Side Effects of Alprazolam are:
- Ataxia
- Anxiety
- Dysarthria, Fatigue
- Constipation
- Drowsiness
- Blurred Vision
- Headache
- Difficulty In Micturition
- Memory Impairment
- Menstrual Disease
- Cognitive Dysfunction
- Diarrhea
- Nervousness, Sedation
- Depression
- Tremor
- Weight Gain
- Weight Loss
- Insomnia
- Decreased Libido
- Increased Appetite
- Irritability
- Skin Rash
- Trouble speaking
- Decreased Appetite

Other side effects include:

- Hyperventilation
- Depersonalization
- Muscle Twitching
- Hypoesthesia
- Hypotension
- Sexual Disorder
- Increased Libido
- Sialorrhea
- Paresthesia

- Dark Urine

Do not take Alprazolam if:

- You have narrow-angle glaucoma.
- You are on medication that inhibits or induces hepatic enzymes CYP3A4 like Ketoconazole, erythromycin or Itraconazole (Sporanox).
- You are allergic to alprazolam or similar medicines (for example, lorazepam (Ativan), Oxazepam (Serax), Diazepam (Valium), Clorazepate (Tranxene), et cetera).
- Have just consumed or are addicted to alcohol or hard drugs.
- You are pregnant (it may cause birth defects or life-threatening withdrawal symptoms in neonates or make the baby dependent on the drug after birth).
- You are below the age of 18.

Alprazolam may cause drowsiness, so it is advisable not to consume it before engaging in a stressful or attention demanding activity.

If any of the following is happening or has happened, in order to ensure that Alprazolam is okay for you, it is imperative to disclose to your doctor:

- a history of depression or suicidal thoughts or behavior
- pregnancy or intention to become pregnant while using the drug
- kidney or liver disease (especially alcoholic liver disease)
- a history of drug or alcohol addiction
- asthma or other breathing disorder
- nursing a baby (the drug can pass through breast-milk)
- open-angle glaucoma
- seizures or epilepsy

- use of a narcotic (opioid) medication.

How to take Alprazolam:

- Take the drug with strict adherence to your doctor's prescription. Strictly obey all the guidelines on your prescription label.
- You may take Alprazolam with or without food.
- Never abuse this medicine by consuming it for a longer time or in larger amounts than prescribed.
- Avoid drinking grapefruit juice or consuming grapefruit products while on this drug as the products may increase blood levels of alprazolam.
- Alprazolam may be habit-forming so misusing it could cause addiction or death. The drug is not for sharing or distribution to any other person, especially if that other person has a history of drug addiction or abuse.
- Drinking alcohol while taking Alprazolam is dangerous because it could enhance respiratory depression and sedation.
- Selling or giving away this medicine without prescription is against the law.
- Do not swallow the orally disintegrating tablet whole. Allow it to dissolve in your mouth without chewing.
- It is not safe to break, cut, crush, or chew Alprazolam when it comes as an extended-release tablet. Always swallow it whole.
- When it is an injection, measure the liquid medicine with the dosing syringe provided.
- Where it is a syrup, measure it with a special dose-measuring cup or medicine spoon. Do not improvise, ask your pharmacist for a dose-measuring device if you do not have one.
- During pregnancy, do not stop using Alprazolam without discussing it with your doctor, which should be as soon as possible.

-   If it appears that the medicine has stopped working well in treating your panic or anxiety symptoms, call your doctor immediately.

Other Considerations

-   To avoid discomforting withdrawal symptoms, do not stop using Alprazolam abruptly. Consult your doctor to know when and how to stop using alprazolam safely.
-   Frequent medical tests are important for persons who use this medicine long-term.
-   If the drug causes depression, talk to your doctor.
-   Storage of the drug should be at room temperature and away from heat and moisture.
-   Keep the drug out of reach of children and pets.
-   Monitor the quantity of medicine used from each new bottle, because being a drug of abuse one should know if anyone is using the medicine improperly or without a medical prescription.
-   If you appear to have grown dependent on or addicted to Alprazolam, talk with your doctor.

DOSAGES

The dosage for this drug is as prescribed by the doctor. But on a general level, adhere to the following guidelines:

For treating anxiety in Adults:

-   Immediate-release tablets or Orally Disintegrating Tablets (ODT): 0.25 to 0.5 mg orally administered 3 times a day
-   Maximum dose: 4 mg/day

For treating Anxiety in elderly or debilitated patients:

-   Immediate-release tablets or Orally Disintegrating Tablets (ODTs): 0.25 mg orally administered 2 or 3 times a day.

Uses:

- For managing Anxiety Disorder or APA DSM-III-R diagnosis of Generalized Anxiety Disorder.
- Short-term relief of symptoms of anxiety.
- Treatment of GAD (Generalized Anxiety Disorder)

For Treating Panic Disorder in Adults;

Immediate-release tablets/ODTs:

- 0.5 mg orally administered 3 times a day
- Maximum dose: 10 mg/day

Extended-release tablets:
-Initial dose: 0.5 to 1 mg orally once a day
-Maintenance dose: 3 to 6 mg orally per day, preferably in the morning
-Maximum dose: 10 mg/day

For treating Panic Disorder in Elderly or Debilitated patients:

Immediate-release tablets/Orally Disintegrating Tablets (ODTs):

- Initial dose: 0.25 mg orally administered 2 or 3 times a day.

Extended-release tablets:
-Initial dose: 0.5 mg orally once a day.

Uses:

- To treat panic disorder, with or without agoraphobia.

Things to Note:

- The drug should be administered in the lowest possible effective dose.
- It is necessary to conduct frequent reassessment of the need for continued treatment.
- Decreasing the daily dosage is limited to no more than 0.5 mg every 3 days, although some

patients may require an even slower reduction of their doses.

- When discontinuing therapy or when decreasing the daily dosage, reduction should be gradual, not abrupt.
- It is okay to increase the dose of extended-release tablets at intervals of 3 to 4 days in increments of no more than 1 mg each day.
- During prescription, it is important to distribute the times of administration as evenly as possible throughout the waking hours.

How Alprazolam works

- Gamma-aminobutyric Acid (GABA) is a neurotransmitter, which blocks impulses between nerve cells in the brain and experts say that low levels of GABA could cause anxiety disorder. Though not exactly sure how Alprazolam works, experts believe that its effects are as a result of its ability to strongly bind to the GABA-benzodiazepine receptor complex, which enhances the affinity for GABA.
- Alprazolam calms and sedates and can therefore be used for the short-term treatment of anxiety and seizure disorders.

c. ESCITALOPRAM OXALATE

It belongs to the SSRI (Selective Serotonin Reuptake Inhibitors) class of drugs. This means that it works by enhancing the restoration of Serotonin in the brain. Other drugs in this category are fluoxetine (Prozac), Sertraline (Zoloft) and Paroxetine (Paxil). It is for treating anxiety as well as depression.

Precautions:

Before taking Escitalopram, let your doctor know if:

- You are allergic to it, to Citalopram, or to any other drug.
- You take diuretics or water pills.

- You have diabetes, Phenylketonuria (PKU) or any other condition that stops you from consuming sugar or aspartame, which is contained in the liquid form of Escitalopram.
- You are pregnant or planning to become pregnant.
- You or any other member of your family has a history of bipolar disorder or manic-depressive disorder.
- You or your family member has a history of suicide attempts or suicide.
- There is a personal or family history of Hyponatremia (Low sodium in the blood), seizures, intestinal ulcers, bleeding problems, Angle-closure glaucoma, liver diseases, and low level of Magnesium or Potassium in the blood.

How to Take Escitalopram Oxalate:
- It is consumed orally.
- A person can consume Escitalopram with or without food, depending on what the doctor says.
- The usual dose is one daily, morning or evening, but doctors may prescribe differently because they consider other factors like conditions to be treated, age and other medications taken.
- The doctor may begin at a lower dose and gradually increase it; do as the doctor says.
- Taking higher doses will not provide a quicker cure in any way; it will worsen your health instead.
- Measure the liquid form of this medicine with a special measuring spoon or measuring cup, using a teaspoon or tablespoon will not provide the accurate dosage.
- Even if you begin to feel perfectly fine, do not stop the dosage suddenly. Instead, consult your doctor to guide you through stopping the dosage. A sudden halt in taking this drug may worsen the condition or cause symptoms like shock, tiredness, mood swings, etc.
- Generally, takes about two weeks to see improvements and four weeks for a total cure. If

your condition does not improve or worsens instead, tell your doctor about it.

WARNING AND SIDE EFFECTS

Usually, the leaflet accompanying the medicine provides this information but usual major side effects are:

- Dizziness
- Tiredness
- Dry mouth
- Drowsiness
- Nausea
- Sleep problems
- Sweating
- SluggishnessThese usually happen in persons taking this drug but if they persist or worsen, contact your doctor. There are other unusual, more serious side effects and once they begin, it is important to conduct your doctor immediately. They are:
- Changes in Libido
- Hallucinations
- Bloody/tarry/black stools
- Red eyes
- Severe nausea
- Irregular or increased heartrate
- Fainting
- Blurred vision
- Twitching Muscles
- Vomit (that resembles coffee grounds)
- Unexplained fever
- Change in Sexual drive
- Diarrhea
- Unusual restlessness
- Rash
- Swollen or itchy throat

THINGS TO NOTE

- Do not share this drug with other people, especially drug addicts or abusers.
- Keep all medical and psychiatric appointments judiciously.

Missed Doses
- As soon as you remember a missed dose, take it but skip it if it is almost time of the next dose, and resume your usual dosage. There is no need to try to catch up by doubling the dose.

Storage

- Store at room temperature.
- Keep away from light and moisture.
- Do not store in the bathroom.
- Keep all medicines away from children and pets.
- Do not flush this drug or any other one down a toilet or a drain unless instructed to do so.
- When this drug expires or has outlived its importance, discard it properly.

d. IMIPRAMINE (TOFRANIL)

It falls in the class of drugs known as Tricyclics. Drugs in this class treat all anxiety disorders except OCD (Obsessive Compulsive Disorder). Another drug in this class is Clomipramine (Anafranil). They serve the same function and have the same side effects. New drugs with lesser side effects are in production and supply so Tricyclics are not in as frequent use as they used to be. They work on the Central Nervous System to enhance certain chemicals in the brain

It usually comes in two forms: capsule and tablet, both of which are consumed orally.

Side Effects:

- Drowsiness
- Vomiting
- Delirium
- Weight gain
- Hallucination
- Blurred vision
- Dry mouth
- Constipation
- Dizziness
- Weakness

When side effects occur, one can control them by either using another Tricyclic or altering the dosage.

If a person consumes Imipramine with or immediately after consuming MOAIs and vice versa, it could lead to seizures or instant death. The shortest safe period between the uses of each drug is 2 weeks. This information is one that requires compulsory disclosure to your physician especially if you are not sure that you have taken any Monoamine Oxidase Inhibitors (MOAIs).

e. ISOCARBOXAZID (MARPLAN)

This drug is a non-selective and irreversible MOAI (Monoamine Oxidase Inhibitors). It belongs to a class of drugs called Hydrazine. Drugs in this class provide treatment for Panic Disorder and Anxiety Disorders (Social Phobia) by increasing the quantity of mood regulating neurotransmitters in the body and acting on other chemicals in the brain. Other MOAIs are Selegiline (Emsam), Phenelzine (Nardil), and Tranylcypromine (Parnate). Just like Tricyclics, MOAIs are old drugs with more side effects than newer drugs.

These drugs, like every drug, have side effects and because of this, MOAIs usually come with some restrictions.

Restrictions

- MOAIs and cheese or red wines are a bad mix.
- They are not taken with certain medications like Ibuprofen, Acetaminophen, SSRIs, medications for colds or allergies, herbal supplements, and some birth control pills.
- If a person has taken other drugs in the MOAI class in the last 14 days, this information must be disclosed before or immediately after the Doctor prescribes Isocarboxazid.

Side Effects

There are severe and less serious side effects of using this drug. The serious side effects include:

- Swelling
- Chest pain
- Sudden, severe headaches
- Jaundice (yellowing of the skin or eyes)
- Rapid heartbeat
- Stiffness in the back and neck
- Nausea
- Fainting
- Sweating
- Vomiting
- Rapid weight gain
- Vision problems like increased sensitivity to light
- Cold sweat
- Irregular heart rate
- Light-headedness

Less serious side effects may include:
- Headache
- Constipation
- Nausea
- Loss of appetite (not common)
- Tremors
- Dry mouth
- Dizziness

- Shaking

When combined with other drugs that increase the levels of the monoamine neurotransmitters like the SSRIs, or with certain foods that are high in dietary amines like aged cheese, MAOIs can produce dangerous increments of monoamine neurotransmitters leading to potentially life-threatening ailments such as Serotonin Syndrome (SS) and Hypertensive crisis. Mixing or using MOAIs with these medications and foods or drinks can also cause low blood pressure and other life-threatening symptoms.

- THERAPY

There is a plethora of therapies that apply to persons suffering from psychological disorders. They are in categories as discussed below:

A. PSYCHOTHERAPY

This is the general name for therapies that are administered for the cure of any psychological disorder, but some authors describe it as a separate procedure. It involves having counselling sessions with a psychologist, psychiatrist, counsellor, social worker or other trained health professional. The sessions are mostly one-one-one sessions and involve discussing the causes, symptoms and possible remedies of anxiety. The professional and the patient also look into the fears associated with the anxious feeling and how the patient can live with them.

B. COGNITIVE-BEHAVIOUR THERAPY (CBT)

It is a one-on-one short-term therapy method used by therapists and counselors to teach people to change their undesirable conduct by changing or improving their thought pattern. It usually lasts from one to twenty sessions, it is problem specific and works towards a relapse of a disorder (in this case, Anxiety and Panic). CBT is based on the theory that it is not actual incidents that cause disorders and other life problems but the interpretation we give to those situations.

Here, the patient learns how to confront their fears and they work on their sensitivity to anxiety triggers and lessen this sensitivity. It teaches a person to focus on reality and detach themselves from the erroneous interpretation they have given to certain events from their past. It teaches patients be rational during panic attacks by making them understand that they're not about to die and they're not having a heart attack but that what they are experiencing is just their body reacting to a situation they are in now. Understanding this brings a level of calmness to the person's mind during the attacks and reduces its severity.

Some common interventions that specialists apply in Cognitive-Behavior Therapy (CBT) are:

- Identify the problem areas.
- Build a cognizance of automatic thoughts.
- Make a distinction between rational and irrational conclusions.
- Stop negative thinking.
- Challenge inherent speculations.
- Analyze situations from various points of view.
- Stop catastrophizing.
- Distinguish reality from hallucinations and delusions.
- Test your perceptions against reality.
- Do not draw hasty conclusions.
- Reshape your thoughts to reflect reality.
- Avoid generalizing (for example, he raped me therefore all men are rapists).
- Examine the validity and utility of a particular thought or line of thoughts.
- Identify distorted beliefs and modify them.
- Enhance awareness of moods.
- Keep a cognitive behavioral diary to record progress.
- Gradually increase exposure to things that are feared.
- Stop the practice of "reading minds" and "fortune telling."
- Stop personalizing and taking blame (the everything is my fault attitude).

- Focus on how things are rather than how you think they should be.
- Describe, accept, and understand rather than judge situations.

It is quite popular and research is in progress to improve on the therapy. In fact, some doctors conduct a brain scan on their Obsessive-Compulsive Disorder (OCD) patients to ascertain how they will respond to CBT. It is the most widely recognized therapy and comes highly recommended.

In some situations, the patient may become dependent on the therapist while some may develop emotional attachments for them, but this is rare.

C. ACCEPTANCE COMMITMENT THERAPY (ACT)

In 2015, a review disclosed that ACT was more effective in treating anxiety, panic and addiction than placebos were. The therapy teaches people not to avoid situations that invoke our fears, but to embrace the unpleasant feelings and learn not to overreact to them. ACT takes us on a path where feelings lead to a better understanding of truth. The goal of this therapy is not to determine difficult situations that cause anxiety; it only tries to be present in life situations and to "move towards Valued Behavior." ACT measures truth through the concept of workability, that is, what works as a step towards what matters (value).

ACT provides a summary of numerous problems we face in life under four major words in the acronym FEAR. The acronym stands for:

- **F**usion with your thoughts
- **E**valuation of experience
- **A**voidance of your experience
- **R**eason-giving for your behavior

It doesn't end there; Acceptance Commitment Therapy tells us that the healthy alternative to FEAR is to **ACT**:

- Accept your reactions and be present
- Choose a valued direction
- Take action

To help patients (clients) achieve psychological flexibility, ACT employs six core principles to wit:

1. **Cognitive Defusion:** Learning ways to reduce the tendency to reckon thoughts, emotions, memories and images. Separating the death instinct from the life instinct and knowing the difference.

2. **Acceptance:** Freely allowing unwanted private experiences (feelings, urges and thoughts) to come and go without fighting them.

3. **Contact with the present moment:** An awareness of the present, experienced with openness, interest, and receptiveness.

4. **The observing self:** Accessing a transcendent sense of self, a continuity of consciousness that is unchanging.

5. **Values:** Discovering the things that matter most to oneself.

6. **Committed action:** Setting valuable or meaningful goals and executing them responsibly.

D. EXPOSURE THERAPY

Exposure therapy is so-called because it involves exposing the patient to the situations, objects or places that instigate a feeling of fear in them. The idea is that through repeated exposures, they will feel an increased sense of control over the feeling and their anxiety will diminish if not extinguish. The process takes one of two forms:

1. The therapist may ask the patient to imagine the scary situation or object and guide him or her through dealing with it.
2. The patient may be made to confront the fearful event, object or place in real life

Exposure therapy can be administered independently, or it may be included as a part of Cognitive Behavioral Therapy.

- SELF-HELP & EXERCISE

There are many things a person can do to avoid or improve the treatment process of anxiety and panic disorders. While these are not expensive, they require commitment and consistency. We have briefly discussed some of these actions and activities below:

I. **The 21-Minute Cure:** Experts say that when a person experiences anxiety, doing a quick-walk, little dance or jog for about 21 minutes is all it takes to calm the nerves.

II. **Drink lots of** Water: Dehydration can cause weakness and hallucination, which could make a person anxious. It is important to keep the body hydrated by consuming water and relevant fluids regularly.

III. **The 4-7-8 Breath:** Dr. Andrew Weils in his book "Spontaneous Happiness" introduced this exercise. It works because it is not possible to hold one's breath and be anxious at the same time. It is also recommendable that one carries out this exercise twice a day.
You can successfully carry out this exercise in three basic steps:
- Exhale completely through your mouth.
- Inhale through your nose and count to four.
- Hold your breath and count to seven.
- Slowly let it out through your mouth for eight counts.

IV. **Healthy Eating:** Breakfast is healthy and important; most people who skip breakfast usually suffer from anxiety disorders. Experts recommend eating a breakfast that is high in protein since it's one of nature's top Choline sources; low levels of Choline could cause increased anxiety.

Omega-3 isn't just good for the heart - it helps protect against anxiety too. Oily cold-water fishes such as mussels, salmon, sardines, and anchovies are rich in Omega-3 fatty acids and good consumption of these can reduce anxiety.

People tend to get more anxious when they are hungry so it is advisable to eat something quick when one begins to get anxious. Eating whole-foods, plenty of leafy greens for folate, plant-based food with seafood and a host of other phytonutrients can help reduce anxiety in the long term.

V. **Quit Catastrophizing:** "Catastrophic thinking" is common during an anxiety attack; the mind selects a lot of horrible possibilities and imagines what would happen if they actually occurred. Instead of dwelling on these thoughts, do something to distract yourself; take deep breaths, read a motivational book, listen to a lively song, take a short walk, etc. and try to focus on the positive aspects of your life.

VI. **Warm up:** A sunny day at the beach, some time by the fire with a hot beverage, a sauna spell, soaking in a hot bath or Jacuzzi etc. anything to keep you warm are all recommended as this could affect the neurotransmitter serotonin, the imbalance of which could cause anxiety.

VII. **Learn to say No:** Set limits on what you can do for yourself and others; learn to say no to requests that will require excessive stress to fulfil.

VIII. **Shinrin-yoku (Forest Bath):** In English, it is a "Walk in the woods." A Japanese study revealed that people who took part in a 20-minute walk in nature had a more noticeable drop in their anxiety levels than when walking in urban areas.

IX. **Exercise:** This is a good antidote for anxiety, both short-term and long-term. Self-exertion can improve self-image and release some brain-chemicals that trigger a good mood.

X. **Support Network:** Talking with a person (like a parent or sibling that can provide support) can go a long way to help. Discussing the cause of anxiety with a loved one can calm anxiety.

XI. **Stress Management:** Life can be overwhelming, especially when you have so much to do and so little time to achieve them; this can make you anxious and if it continues, may cause panic or anxiety disorder.
Making a comfortable and realistic To-do list each day, coming up with more enjoyable ways to carry out tasks, and concentrating on how far you have come rather than how much more there is to do can reduce stress. Reduced stress means reduced anxiety and with time, the triggers will diminish and probably disappear.

PART 5: CONCLUSION, RECOMMENDATIONS AND DISCLAIMER

5.0 CONCLUSION

This may sound weird, but the good thing about life is that no matter how badly you think you're doing, there's someone out there doing a lot worse. What's even weirder is that they aren't half as worried as you are. Another thing is that there really is no novel condition as far as the world is concerned; therefore, your problem is not peculiar to you. Many other people have suffered it or are currently in it, even if you don't know it.

Life is mysterious. It has its vicissitudes and this mix is what makes it even more interesting. The truth about life is that no matter how rosy your neighbor's garden may seem, the thorns exist therein and they are not blunt. There is no perfect life and the earlier we accept this, the better. Many have lost their lives to panic attacks; many have become slaves to anxiety either because they're trying to meet some flimsy standard set by society or because they have refused to let go of negative past experiences. We are our own boss. Nobody has the right to tell you how much you ought to have achieved at a particular age or time in your life; the life is yours. Thus, while it's okay to aim for greatness, it's wrong to measure your achievements based on what another person has achieved. It's unhealthy to beat yourself up over little things like "My college rival got married before me, she got that new position I was competing against her for," and other little things that we dwell on, which make us anxious about what tomorrow holds.

This book has provided an insight into what anxiety and panic are, the causes and symptoms, at what stage they become disorders, how to prevent them and how to overcome them. It also tells us that there are people experiencing this too and so we shouldn't feel ashamed that we have to handle this. The book tells us of survivors, not for entertainment purposes but as a way to assure us that just like everything else in life, this phase will surely pass, but there are things we must do if we must survive them.

5.1 RECOMMENDATIONS

Research shows that most patients of anxiety and panic disorders usually resort to self-medication when they self-diagnose themselves with the disorder. We should all understand that treatment varies for every type of disorder and further varies for each type of anxiety disorder.

Furthermore, taking the wrong medication could bring about worse problems beyond emotions and psychology. It may lay the necessary foundation for terminal illnesses and other painful heath conditions. It is not productive to solve a problem by creating another one, so self-diagnosis is inherently wrong.

There are those who stop their medications immediately when they notice some form of improvement. The effect of this is that side effects will manifest as symptoms and since the patient may not know that these symptoms are because of suddenly quitting the medication, they begin to cure the symptoms one after the other or cure the diseases they think the symptoms suggest.

The author thus recommends the following:

1. Do not diagnose yourself of any medical condition for any reason.
2. Ensure you follow the directives given by your physician.
3. If you start reacting to the medicine, notify your physician immediately.
4. No medicine works on everybody in the same way, so what worked on your sister or other relative may worsen your situation, so do not self-medicate.
5. If you decide to combine your medication with a therapy, notify the doctor and the therapist of the therapy and the drugs.

6. If you have a reason to stop your medication or start another one (even if it is for a different ailment), consult with your doctor and get his consent.
7. If you become pregnant in the course of your treatment, let your physician know of the development and inform your gynecologist of the treatment.
8. Stop assumptions concerning what works best for you; ascertain everything with your physician.
9. The fact that your symptoms are listed on medical blogs as indicative of an ailment does not mean that you are suffering from that ailment; always confer with a professional.

5.2 DISCLAIMER

THIS BOOK DOES NOT REPLACE THE NEED TO SEEK MEDICAL ADVICE FROM A HEALTH CARE PROFESSIONAL

The information, including but not limited to, text, graphics, images and other material available in this book are for your *information* only. The author does not intend that the book become a substitute for professional medical advice, diagnosis or treatment. Therefore, no one should construe the contents of this book as medical advice or instruction. No reader should engage in any action or inaction based solely on the contents of or the information in this book.

The author does not recommend or endorse any tests, opinions, physicians, products, procedures, studies or other information mentioned in this book. Therefore, all readers are advised unequivocally to consult appropriate health professionals on any matter relating to their health and well-being.

Every piece of information and opinion expressed herein are believed by the author to be accurate, based on the best judgement available to the author. Therefore, any reader who fails to take the recommendations made and consequently omits to consult with the appropriate health authorities assumes the liability for any injuries or damage caused by such omission.

In addition, the information and opinions expressed herein do not necessarily reflect the views of every contributor to the writing and publishing of this book. The author acknowledges the possibility of occasional differences in opinion and welcomes the exchange of different viewpoints at any time. The publisher shall not be held accountable for errors or omissions discovered in the course of reading this book.

BIBLIOGRAPHY

Books

American Psychiatric Association (2013). Diagnostic and Statistical Manual of Mental Disorders (5th ed.). Washington, D.C.: American Psychiatric Association

American Psychiatric Association (4th ed.) (2000) Diagnostic and Statistical Manual of Mental Disorders, Text Revision (DSM-IV-TR) Washington, DC: American Psychiatric Association.

Hayes, S. C., Strosahl, K. D. & Wilson, K. G. (2012). *Acceptance and Commitment Therapy: The Process and Practice of Mindful Change* (2 ed.). New York: Guilford Press. p. 240.

Hayes, Steven C.; Strosahl, Kirk D.; Wilson, Kelly G. (2012). *Acceptance and Commitment Therapy: The Process and Practice of Mindful Change* (2 ed.). New York: Guilford Press. p. 240.

Nelson-Jones, R. (2009). Theory and Practice of Counseling and Therapy. (4th ed.) London: Sage Publications.

Robert A. Williams, MD; "Brain Basics: A Biological Approach to Human Behavior", Biological Psychiatry Institute, Phoenix.

Online Sources

Acceptance and Commitment Therapy. (n.d.). In *Wikipedia*. Retrieved May 29, 2018, from https://en.wikipedia.org/wiki/Acceptance_and_commitment_therapy

Amsterdam J.D., Li Y., Soeller I., Rockwell K., Mao J. J., & Shults J. (2009, August). A Randomized, Double-blind, Placebo-controlled Trial of Oral Matricaria recutita (Chamomile) Extract Therapy for Generalized Anxiety Disorder. *J Clin Psychopharmacol.* 29(4):378-82. Retrieved from https://www.ncbi.nlm.nih.gov/pubmed/19593179

Andrew Weil, MD (2011) *Spontaneous Happiness* [Kindle Version]. Retrieved from https://www.amazon.com/Spontaneous-Happiness-Andrew-Weil/dp/0316129445

Anxiety and Depression Association of America, Understanding the Facts, Suicide and Prevention [Blog Post]. Retrieved from https://adaa.org/understanding-anxiety/suicide#

Biological Psychiatry Institute (n.d.). Panic Disorders. *Beyond Blue*. Retrieved from https://www.beyondblue.org.au/the-facts/anxiety/types-of-anxiety
Center for Clinical Interventions. (n.d.) Coping with Physical Alarms: Exposure Part 1 (PDF) Retrieved from http://www.cci.health.wa.gov.au/docs/Panic-09_Exposure-1.pdf

Takeuchi T, Hasegawa M, Ikeda M, Hayashi R, Tomiyama G, Nemoto T, Hoshino K. (1992 March). Four Clinical Types of Panic Disorders. Chiba Japan: Department of Psychiatry, Ichihara Hospital, Teikyo University School of Medicine. Jpn J Psychiatry Neurol. 46(1):37-44. Retrieved from https://www.ncbi.nlm.nih.gov/pubmed/1635333#

Kamenov K., Twomey C., Cabello M, Prina A. M., Ayuso-Mateos J. L. (2017 February). The Efficacy of Psychotherapy, Pharmacotherapy and their Combination on Functioning and Quality of Life in Depression: a Meta-analysis. *Psychol Med.* 47(3) 414-425. Retrieved from https://www.ncbi.nlm.nih.gov/pmc/articles/PMC5244449/

Kennedy D. O., Little W & Scholey A. B. (2004, July - August). Attenuation of Laboratory-induced Stress in Humans after Acute Administration of Melissa officinalis (Lemon Balm) [Blog Post]. Retrieved from https://www.ncbi.nlm.nih.gov/pubmed/15272110

Kohlenberg, R., Hayes S. & Tsai, M. (1993). Radical Behavioral Psychotherapy: Two Contemporary Examples. *Clinical Psychology Review*, *13*(6) 579-592. Retrieved from https://www.sciencedirect.com/science/article/pii/02727358 9390047P?via%3Dihub

Mark S. G.. Good News about Depression. Biological Psychiatry Institute: Phoenix.
Medical News Today (2017 November 12). Treatments for Anxiety [Blog Post]. Retrieved from https://www.medicalnewstoday.com/info/anxiety/anxiety-treatments.php

Newman, D. J., Cragg, G. M. & Snader K. M. (2003). Natural Products as Sources of New Drugs over the Period 1981–2002. *PubMed, 66*(7) 1022–1037. Retrieved from https://www.ncbi.nlm.nih.gov/pubmed/12880330

Nootriment. (n.d.). Valerian Root for Anxiety, Stress, Panic Attacks and Social Anxiety. Retrieved from https://nootriment.com/valerian-root-for-anxiety/

Nuphorin. (n.d.). 21 Herbs for Anxiety and Panic Attacks. Retrieved from https://www.nuphorin.com/21-herbs-for-anxiety/

Srivastava JK, Shankar E, & Gupta S. (2003, November 1). "Chamomile: A herbal medicine of the past with bright future," Mol Med Rep. *3*(6) 895-901. Retrieved from https://www.ncbi.nlm.nih.gov/pmc/articles/PMC2995283/

Takeuchi T, Hasegawa M., Ikeda M, Hayashi R., Tomiyama G., Nemoto T., & Hoshino K. (1992, March) Four Clinical Types of Panic Disorders. *.Jpn J Psychiatry Neurol, 46*(1) 37-44. Retrieved from https://www.ncbi.nlm.nih.gov/pubmed/1635333#

Weissman M. M., Klerman G.L., Markowitz J. S., & Ouellette R. (1989, November 2). Suicidal Ideation and Suicide Attempts in Panic Disorder and Attacks. *N Engl J Med.*, *321*(18) 1209–1214. Retrieved from https://www.ncbi.nlm.nih.gov/pubmed/2797086

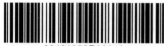

Made in the USA
Columbia, SC
15 June 2019